Praise for the Miriam Bender Exercise Program

"This extraordinary program must be brought to the forefront as a beneficial approach for eliminating ADHD symptoms."

—Pamela Bandy, M.S., OTR, occupational therapist,
Riley Hospital for Children

"I have personally seen the benefits of this breakthrough procedure not only with my patients but also with my seven-year-old son and my seventy-seven-year-old mother."

—Robert C. Prather, D.C., DABCI, LAC

"This program has my enthusiastic support. Sufficient crawling is essential for efficient visual and perceptual motor development."

—Raymond F. Parker, O.D., Fellow,
American Academy of Optometry

"The children served in my occupational therapy practice, their families, and I are grateful to Dr. O'Dell and Dr. Cook for making Dr. Bender's work accessible! This approach is effective, simple, and easily done with commitment and consistency."

—Amy Beaupre, M.S., OTR

"In my nursing practice and as a parent, I have seen the Miriam Bender program make dramatic improvements in children and adults."

—Janet DeFelice, B.S., R.N.

"This program is known to me personally and professionally to ease stress and frustration, bring harmony to the family unit, and improve academic success."

—Sandra A. Zimmerman, LCSW, LMHC, M.S., R.N.

Stopping ADHD

Stopping ADHD

A Unique and Proven Drug-Free Program for Treating ADHD in Children and Adults

Nancy E. O'Dell, Ph.D.
Patricia A. Cook, Ph.D.

Previously published as
Stopping Hyperactivity

Avery
a Member of Penguin Group (USA) Inc.
New York

Neither the publisher nor the authors are engaged in rendering professional advice or services to the individual reader. The ideas, procedures, and suggestions contained in this book are not intended as a substitute for consulting with your physician. All matters regarding your health require medical supervision. Neither the authors nor the publisher shall be liable or responsible for any loss or damage allegedly arising from any information or suggestion in this book.

While the authors have made every effort to provide accurate telephone numbers and Internet addresses at the time of publication, neither the publisher nor the authors assume any responsibility for errors or for changes that occur after publication.

Most Avery books are available at special quantity discounts for bulk purchase for sales promotions, premiums, fund-raising, and educational needs. Special books or book excerpts also can be created to fit specific needs. For details, write Penguin Group (USA) Inc. Special Markets, 375 Hudson Street, New York, NY 10014.

AVERY

a member of
Penguin Group (USA) Inc.
375 Hudson Street
New York, NY 10014
www.penguin.com

Library of Congress Cataloging-in-Publication Data

O'Dell, Nancy.
    Stopping ADHD : a unique and proven drug-free program for treating ADHD in children and adults / Nancy E. O'Dell, Patricia A. Cook.
        p.   cm.
    Includes bibliographical references and index.
    ISBN 1-58333-197-2
    1. Attention-deficit hyperactivity disorder—Etiology.   2. Attention-deficit hyperactivity disorder—Exercise therapy.   3. Abnormal reflexes.   I. Cook, Patricia.   II. Title.

RJ506.H9O338   2004   2004046131
618.92'8589—dc22

Printed in the United States of America
10   9   8   7   6   5   4   3   2   1

Interior photos of exercises by Thomas Cook
Book design by Lovedog Studio

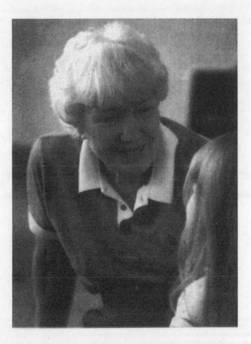

We joyously dedicate this book
to the memory of Dr. Miriam L. Bender.

Acknowledgments

Together: We are truly appreciative of the support we have received from friends and colleagues at the University of Indianapolis and at Purdue, and from our personal and professional friends over the years. We thank the Wilen sisters, who graciously directed us to Rudy Shur, without whom the first edition of our book might never have been published. Many thanks to our editor, Dara Stewart, for her unwavering, steadfast support and perseverance in following our additions, deletions, and arrows in the publication of this second edition. Thanks, also, to our copy editor, Kathleen Stahl, for her painstaking attention to detail. Thanks to Shirley Bigna, Kelly Cook, and David Parker for help in research; to Elizabeth Clark and Beth Kiggins for computer support; to Robert Hendren for legal assistance; to our three "model children": Kelsey Gray, John Andrew Clark, and Charlie Newport; and to Tom Cook, cinematographer, for an outstanding job. Together, of course, we pay our homage to Miriam Bender, without whose vision and support we would never have known about the symmetric tonic neck reflex. Above all, we thank God for enabling us to be involved in this special work.

Pat: How does one thank family and friends for continuous support? Putting them in the section called "Acknowledgments" is insufficient, but at least it's in print. My love and appreciation for a lifetime of support go to Art Cook; to my sons and their families—Tom and Kelly,

Benjamin and Walter; Kevin and Pam, Cal and Lily—to Raymond and Corinne Parker and to Ray and Bonnie and all my wonderful Parker nieces and nephews; to Jeanne; to Betty Lou and her family; to the Powells; to Judy Ramsey; to all my cousins; and to the families attached to all these loved ones; to all those teachers who inspired and directed me; to the Lunch Bunch, the Marian and Lourdes Groups; to students and teaching friends and personal friends; to all who have been interested and encouraging. Thanks to Marcia Miller and Suzie Douglass for sending pertinent items from many sources. My part in this book is dedicated to Miriam and Nancy, and especially to Art.

Nancy: For their love and unwavering support, I am eternally grateful to my beloved family, especially my parents, Malcolm and Eleanor Woodworth; my brother, Malcolm Woodworth; my sister and brother-in-law, Susan and Charles Bravard; my son, Greg, and his family Tawnya and Kayla; my daughter, Beth, and her family, John, John Andrew, and Mary Elizabeth; all of my dear aunts and uncles, especially Aunt Clemie, and my grandparents; my devoted pets, Digger, Flanner, Buchanan, Mrs. Beasley, Old Yeller, Big Handsome Boy, Pretty Little Girl, Chessie, Shadow, Tigger, Tarzan, Figaro, and Bootsie; other loving relatives, teachers, colleagues, students, and friends. Special love and appreciation for this book go to Pat, Miriam, and my beloved mother.

Contents

Foreword   *xv*
Preface   *xvii*
Introduction   1

Part One
What Is the Real Problem?   7

1. **The Real Problem**   9
    The Behaviors of ADHD Children
    The Discomfort of ADHD Children
    The Source of Discomfort

2. **The Symmetric Tonic Neck Reflex**   15
    Early Childhood Development
    The Role of the Symmetric Tonic Neck Reflex
    The Importance of Crawling to the Maturation
       of the STNR
    Reasons for Not Crawling Long Enough
       and Properly: Genetic and Environmental
    A Consequence of the "Back to Sleep" Movement:
       Not Crawling Long Enough and Properly
    The Consequences of Not Crawling Long Enough
       and Properly

3.   **Looking for Clues to the Real Problem**   33
      Medical (Mis)Diagnosis and (Mis)Treatment
      STNR Children in Favorite Positions—
         Postural Clues
      Body Language as a Postural Clue

4.   **Psychological Consequences**
      of an Immature STNR   54
      Poor Peer Relationships
      Low Self-Esteem
      Frustration, Avoidance, and Aggression
      Inflexibility

Part Two
How to Work Around the Real Problem   65

5.   **School Problems**   69
      Comfort and Attention Span
      Writing (Dysgraphia)
      Reading and Spelling (Dyslexia)
      Math (Dyscalculia)
      Art and Music
      Physical Education
      Accelerated and Enrichment Classes

6.   **Sports Problems**   99
      Baseball
      Basketball
      Volleyball
      Football
      Swimming
      Wrestling
      Hockey
      Soccer

Skiing
Golf and Tennis
Summary

7. **Problems at Home**   *110*
Mealtime
Homework
After-School Fatigue or Overactivity
Music Lessons
Family Recreation, Games, and
   Television

8. **Problems in Public Settings**   *119*
Traveling
Restaurants
Religious Services
The Doctor's Office
Barbershops and Beauty Salons
Spectator Events

Part Three
How to Solve the Real Problem   *129*

9. **The STNR Exercises**   *133*
Getting Ready
General Directions
The Exercises
How to Know When the Reflex Is Matured

10. **Exercises to Follow the Reflex Program**   *177*
Gross Motor Exercises
Fine Motor Exercises

Conclusion   *185*

Appendixes   187

   A. To Drug or Not to Drug   187
     Abridged Glossary of Medical Terms
   B. Questions and Answers   205
   C. Results of a Study Putting the STNR Program
     in Action in an Elementary School   221

Glossary   231
References   233
Index   239
About the Authors   247

Foreword

How many times have you heard or asked,

"Why can't this child sit still?"
"Why isn't this child's handwriting legible?"
"Why does this child refuse to do simple homework?"

This book presents a unique, effective, and drug-free approach for solving many learning and behavioral problems. This solution can make the lives of millions of children, parents, and teachers happier, easier, and more fulfilling.

My years as a clinician at the Purdue Achievement Center for Children had reinforced my conviction that academic success is significantly based on early motor development. While I was doing my original research at Purdue University on remediation for inadequate motor development, I was fortunate to work with two graduate students, who are now dear friends.

Nancy and Pat enthusiastically embraced my theory and incorporated my remedial exercises into their own clinical practice. These two dedicated teacher-clinicians have successfully worked with many children and adults for more than twenty-five years. Now they are sharing the theory and implementation of my program in their book.

Nancy and Pat, now full professors at the University of Indianapolis, have given numerous presentations to enthusiastic audiences at national and international conferences, including the First International Symposium for Special Education in Beijing, China. This book, written for parents and teachers, now makes Pat and Nancy's clinical and educational experiences available to the world.

I am proud of and excited about their new book and their devoted continuation of my work. It was a fortunate day when we met. I give them, as I always have, my blessings and my thanks. Into their capable and loving hands I gladly pass the torch.

Miriam L. Bender, Ph.D.
Professor Emeritus
Georgia Southern University
Statesboro, Georgia

(March 13, 1908–October 5, 2002)

Preface

As English teachers more than thirty years ago, we constantly wondered why some of our bright students experienced so many academic and behavioral difficulties. In searching for explanations, we encountered numerous descriptions of symptoms such as "short attention span," "nervous energy" (now called Attention-Deficit Hyperactivity Disorder, or ADHD), and learning disabilities. While traditional treatments for these symptoms may have reduced the severity of some behaviors, no traditional treatment has effectively addressed the basic cause of the problem.

The lives of millions of children and adults continue to be more difficult and frustrating than need be because of a little-known reflex that can make merely trying to sit still a laborious, stressful task. It is our hope that *Stopping ADHD: A Unique and Proven Drug-Free Program for Treating ADHD in Children and Adults* will make this reflex, the Symmetric Tonic Neck Reflex, far better known and will broaden public understanding of the ways in which improper or insufficient crawling in infancy leads to behavioral and academic problems in later life.

Stopping ADHD: A Unique and Proven Drug-Free Program for Treating ADHD in Children and Adults is a continuation of the inspirational work of Miriam L. Bender, P.T., Ph.D. Dr. Bender's service as a physical therapist in the armed forces during World War II provided her with a concentrated wealth of experience concerning the workings of the human body. Retiring at the age of sixty-two with the rank of lieutenant colonel, she entered Purdue University and earned a doctorate in 1971. With her background in physical therapy, she extended Dr. Newell Kephart's studies of human movement from the gross-motor level down to the basic-reflex level.

In 1970, we were privileged to begin working with Dr. Bender at Purdue. Dr. Bender offered a revolutionary yet simple explanation of a major cause of attention deficit and hyperactivity. Her explanation was logical, and her remediation program produced significant improvement. This honored professor of education had made a remarkable discovery, one that could dramatically affect the lives of millions of children and their parents.

Dr. Bender's work with learning disabled children was so progressive, innovative, and successful that we enthusiastically and devotedly "took up the torch" and began to implement her approach in the Indianapolis area. After earning our doctorates at Purdue University, we established the Miriam Bender Diagnostic Center in her honor. Our clinic in Indianapolis, Indiana, is the only one of its kind. Here, we put Dr. Bender's theories into practice, emphasizing the reflex-motor facets of learning and behavior. For more than thirty years, we have effectively used Dr. Bender's remediation techniques in eliminating ADHD behavior and learning disabilities in children and adults.

For a number of years, we presented this new approach on our television program, *Info for Living,* and at many national and international conventions, including the First International Symposium for Special Education in Beijing, China. We continue to give presentations around the world.

After many years of successful clinical work and hundreds of presentations in the United States and abroad, we thought it was time to bring the news of our work to a larger audience. Our first edition, *Stopping Hyperactivity: A New Solution,* elaborated on Dr. Bender's theory and rationale. We wrote that book to provide both professionals and parents with a clear understanding of a major cause of ADHD behaviors and numerous other learning disabilities. We also presented the techniques developed to eradicate the underlying cause of these problems. We are pleased that our first edition has been translated into three additional languages—Chinese, German and Czech.

This second edition contains three totally new sections, as well as elaborations and revisions. One new section presents, in understandable language, the adverse side effects of the drugs most commonly prescribed for ADHD therapy. A question-and-answer section shares the questions and comments we have received via letters, phone calls, and e-mails from around the world. The third new section reports the positive results of our research study in implementing the STNR exercises at a local grade school. We have significantly elaborated on the SIDS–Back to Sleep Campaign and its relationship to the STNR. We have also made revisions in the time frame in the STNR exercises.

We are certain that this new edition provides important new information and enhances the implementation of the STNR exercise program. (A supplementary video or DVD that demonstrates the STNR exercises is available. See p. 186 for contact information.)

"Although the world is full of suffering, it is also full of the overcoming of it."

—HELEN KELLER

"God, give us grace to accept with serenity the things that cannot be changed, courage to change the things that should be changed, and the wisdom to distinguish one from the other."

—REINHOLD NIEBUHR

"The happiness of a child should never be sacrificed for educational traditions."

—NANCY E. O'DELL AND PATRICIA A. COOK

Introduction

For more than three decades, psychologists, medical doctors, and educators have attempted to overcome attention-deficit/hyperactivity disorder* (ADHD), and a host of other learning disabilities by treating the overt symptoms of these conditions. Although some of the treatments employed may have helped to diminish some behaviors, none of them has done anything to affect the root cause of these problems.

Dr. Miriam L. Bender's research indicates that many children experience behavioral and academic difficulties because of an immature symmetric tonic neck reflex. Although the symmetric tonic neck reflex occurs naturally in the normal development of children, if this reflex stays at an immature level, it can greatly interfere with coordination tasks.

The Symmetric Tonic Neck Reflex (STNR) operates in response to the position of the head in relation to the body: when the head is tilted back, tension is increased in the muscles that straighten the elbows and those that bend the hips and knees. When the head is bent

---

* *The Diagnostic and Statistical Manual,* 4th edition (DSM-IV-TR), published by the American Psychiatric Association, refers to the previously named ADD/ADHD condition with a new term, Attention-Deficit/Hyperactivity Disorder. The use of an abbreviation is currently in a state of flux, with the most common usage, as of this writing, being ADHD.

forward, tension is increased in the muscles that bend the elbows and those that straighten the hips and knees. Essentially, the three body units—neck, arms, and legs—are "tied together" by the reflex, so that movement in one area *automatically* produces a change in the muscular tension of the other two areas.

In normal development, the STNR reaches its peak strength during the sixth to eighth month of the infant's life. Through proper and sufficient (at least six months) crawling, the STNR should be appropriately diminished in strength by the time the child is two years of age. Retention of STNR activity beyond the age of two at a level that modifies voluntary movement is considered to be "immature," or abnormal, reflex development. The educational implications of abnormal STNR activity can be quite complex and far-reaching. Its presence in the immature state controls the pattern of muscular tension in the child's arms and legs in relation to the head movements; movement of any one of the three involved body parts elicits the reflex response in the other two parts. These involuntary movements interfere with the child's gaining control over the body—that is, the body still controls the child. All movements that the child makes must be performed within the constricting influence of the STNR. The child must almost consciously attend to even simple motor acts.

The immature reflex generally hampers the production of rhythmic, coordinated movement and specifically interferes with the postures generally required for reading and writing.

An immature STNR makes it very difficult for the child to sit at a desk in the "correct sitting position," with elbows and hips bent at the same time. Under the influence of the reflex, the neck and elbows want to straighten in opposition to the bending of the legs, and vice versa. Consequently, when the child bends his or her arms to write or hold a book for reading, the legs tend to straighten. Frequently such children sit slouched down with legs stretched out in front of them. Many teachers consider this position "bad for the spine," indicative of laziness, and a hindrance to the child's work. What these teachers do not realize is that this position is actually a comfortable position for the child with an immature STNR because the arms and neck are not "fighting" with the position of hips and legs.

When not allowed to sit in a slouched position, the STNR child may frequently become a "foot sitter," sitting in the chair with feet and legs tucked under the child's body. This position "locks" the feet down so that the arms and neck can bend while the legs are also bent. Another favorite posture for such children involves hooking the feet around the legs of the chair.

Research (Bender 1971) indicates that approximately 75 percent of the children with learning disabilities have an immature STNR as a contributing factor. This means that for many children who are failing spelling, the basic problem might be more a difficulty with writing than actually with spelling. Many STNR children can pass a spelling test if they are allowed to do it orally rather than having to write the words. In arithmetic, STNR children frequently experience more trouble and expend more energy in copying the problems from a book or from a chalkboard than in comprehending the concepts and computations. These children frequently will do the first parts of their assignments correctly but then will either not finish at all or will just put any answer on the paper in order to hand in a "finished" product. As time passes and they experience failure again and again, they tend to avoid written work and often appear lazy and uninterested in their schoolwork.

Many children with immature STNR are diagnosed as ADHD because of the difficulty in maintaining attention and in sitting still for long periods of time in the "proper sitting position." They may get up and sit down again repeatedly in order to relieve the tension caused by the reflex. These children usually have poor penmanship, write laboriously, form letters poorly, and hold a pencil or pen in a rigid or awkward manner. Every shift of the arm while writing also causes a change in the tension in the neck and hips. Consequently, these children generally write in a quite constricted, restricted, and cramped style and position to avoid muscular changes. Copying from the board to a paper on the desk is an especially difficult task, because the child has to contend with positional changes in the neck and arm and the reflex effects of these changes. Children who combat these problems may choose to write laboriously, almost drawing their letters. While the finished product may look good, the time and effort expended are disproportionately high. Even if a paper looks well done, if the production of the paper takes significantly longer than it does for other children, the action is inefficient. Dr. Bender (1997) estimates that STNR children use at least ten times as much energy as do children without these problems. Not all academic problems result from an immature STNR; however, many academic problems are compounded by this reflex's interference.

We have tried to make all the information in this book as easily understandable as possible. The book is divided into three parts. Part One, "What Is the Real Problem?," explains what the underlying problem is, how it can be detected, and the impact it has on a child's behavior and learning.* It also examines the frequent misdiagnosis and mistreatment of the real problem. Part Two, "How to Work Around the Real Problem," provides solutions for working around these behavior problems. While these solutions will not cure the behavior, they will allow a parent or teacher to cope more successfully with the child on a day-to-day basis. Part Three, "How to Solve the Real Problem," offers a group of daily exercises specifically designed to eliminate the root cause of the problem.

We believe that changing the current approaches to remediation of ADHD, and learning disabilities will not be easy. We expect to hear a good deal of criticism from those who would rather keep things as they are. Nevertheless, no matter how great the criticism may be, there can be no greater defense of a method than the experience of its success, and from years of experience we can tell you that our simple, drug-free program *works*. "There are no adverse side effects and the benefits last a lifetime." (Stevens 2000, p. 162)

---

* If this problem is not solved in childhood, it persists into adulthood. Many adults suffer from the effects of an immature STNR. Because adults are allowed to stand up or slouch or move around more freely than children, the problem has frequently not been identified in adults. However, in recent years, the diagnosis of adult ADHD has significantly increased (*Audio-Digest,* 2003). While the major thrust of this book discusses children, be advised that these same descriptions and sufferings apply to adults as well. The solution in this book for these problems is *equally effective* for adults as for children.

It is our hope, then, that this book will allow you, our readers, to judge for yourselves just how easy it is to overcome these learning disabilities when the root cause is properly diagnosed and then corrected. Dr. Bender's work has made and continues to make the lives of countless thousands of children and adults easier and happier. Anyone who benefits from the concepts in this book has Dr. Miriam L. Bender to thank.

PART ONE

What Is the Real Problem?

Does your child or anyone you know display the following behaviors?

- squirming
- sitting "inappropriately"
- getting up frequently
- losing attention quickly
- daydreaming frequently
- writing poorly
- writing laboriously
- reversing letters or numbers
- moving awkwardly or clumsily
- avoiding athletics
- developing athletic skills slowly

If the answer is, "Yes," and your child has been labeled with attention-deficit/hyperactivity disorder (ADHD) or any other learning disability, we think you will find this book of great interest. Within it, we present compelling evidence that effectively challenges the current medical diagnosis and treatment of ADHD and many other behavioral and learning problems. If you have found that your life is dominated by the constant disruptive behavior of a child, we will provide you with a simple, logical, and accurate explanation of the real causes of this behavior, and we will offer you effective methods to eliminate behavior problems *without the use of drugs.*

We have addressed the most common disruptive behaviors that occur in children diagnosed with ADHD—difficulty sitting still in an "appropriate" position and paying attention. These sitting and attention difficulties are caused by a child's being extremely uncomfortable, and this extreme discomfort has a real, physical basis.

We present a new and unique explanation and solution for most of the problems that have plagued children since schools made "Sit still!" and "Sit up straight!" and "Pay attention!" become a way of life.

1. The Real Problem

Many children seem unable to sit still, pay attention, or function normally in school, home, and community situations where controlled behavior is expected. Parents of these children may find that their lives are dominated by the child's constant disruptive behavior. Frequently, these children are labeled with attention-deficit/hyperactivity disorder (ADHD) or some other learning disability. There is a simple, logical, and accurate explanation of the real cause of this behavior: these children are extremely uncomfortable, and their extreme discomfort has a real, physical basis.

The Behaviors of ADHD Children

The most common disruptive behavior that occurs in children diagnosed with ADHD is difficulty sitting still in an "appropriate" position. They squirm, sit "inappropriately," get up frequently, lose attention, and daydream. In addition, these children often exhibit poor handwriting, reverse letters and numbers as they write, and find the act of writing a great struggle. They often move awkwardly or clumsily; consequently, they may avoid athletics or develop athletic skills slowly.

Not Just a Problem for Children

If this problem is not solved in childhood, it persists into adulthood. Many adults suffer from the effects of an immature STNR. Because adults are allowed to stand up or slouch or move around more freely than children, the problem has frequently not been identified in adults. However, in recent years, the diagnosis of adult ADHD has significantly increased (*Audio-Digest,* 2003). While the major thrust of this book discusses children, be advised that these same descriptions and sufferings apply to adults as well. The solution in this book for these problems is *equally effective* for adults as for children.

School Behaviors

Most teachers assume that sitting still, in a socially acceptable position, is comfortable, easy to do, and relaxing. However, if sitting "appropriately" is so easily managed, then why do some children consistently resist this "relaxing" position? If sitting appropriately is so easy, why is "Keeping Johnny in His Seat" the usual goal of behavior-modification programs? Teachers struggle continually to keep some children seated at all, much less "appropriately." Frequently, teachers spend more time telling children to stay in their seats, sit still, sit up straight, and pay attention than they do teaching reading, writing, and arithmetic. Do some of these comments sound familiar?

- "Why can't these kids sit still?"
- "I spend half my time just trying to keep Johnny in his seat."
- "The work Janie does is good, but I have to keep after her all the time to get her to finish it."
- "The poor kid has missed three recesses this week trying to get all the work done."
- "He squirms around so much he misses half the directions."
- "If he would just try a little harder . . ."

These children can't sit still, can't stay put, can't stop squirming, and can't pay attention no matter how hard they try, because *they are uncomfortable*.

Home Behaviors

Equally frustrating are some home situations. Most parents, like most teachers, assume that sitting is comfortable, easy to do, and relaxing. Unfortunately, the children who cannot meet the demand to sit appropriately in school have the same difficulties at home. Consequently, these children hear the negative comments of their teachers at school repeated by their parents at home.

- "Why can't you sit up at the dinner table?"
- "How many times do I have to tell you not to sit on your legs?"
- "Don't do your homework lying on the floor. Why do you think we bought you a desk?"
- "We just can't take you to church anymore. You're all over the pew."
- "People must think we don't discipline you at all. You're so antsy."
- "Why can't you pay attention when I'm talking to you?"
- "You just don't try hard enough!"

These children can't sit still, can't stay put, can't stop squirming, and can't pay attention no matter how hard they try, because *they are uncomfortable*.

The Discomfort of ADHD Children

What do we mean when we say that a child is uncomfortable? To begin with, there are varying degrees of discomfort—from mild to extreme discomfort. Try to imagine the discomfort of sitting a little too long on a straight-backed, cushionless wooden chair. The longer you sit, the more uncomfortable you become, fidgeting and shifting your weight from side to side in an attempt to release your muscular tension.

Now imagine that you are told you must sit in that chair for an indeterminate length of time. As the hours go by, your body begins to ache. Your muscles beg to be stretched. You find no relief in any sitting position you try. As more time passes, these feelings intensify. Minutes seem like hours. Time becomes distorted. Someone barks an order to you, but it is hard to focus on what he is asking you to do. In order to cope with the discomfort, you try to think of other things—friends, family, vacations, anything to take your mind off what you are feeling. What you are experiencing now is extreme discomfort, a degree of discomfort often used by interrogation experts as torture.

Some children do not have to sit in a chair for hours to feel so uncomfortable. Discomfort begins to work on them within minutes of sitting down. For these children, discomfort is not an unusual circumstance, but a part of their everyday experience, a condition that permeates their world. Because this discomfort has always been with them, they do not know that what they are experiencing is unusual—that there is a problem. They assume that everyone else is also uncomfortable, and they wonder how other people are able to sit still and get their work done quickly. As parents and teachers, we have misinterpreted the behavior that uncomfortable children exhibit. Without knowing what to look for, we have been blind to the obvious. Once we know what to look for, the real problem becomes apparent.

If you question the kind and degree of discomfort that these children feel, we would like you to perform the exercise we call "The Spelling Bee" (see the inset on page 13). It should give you an inkling of what a child with this problem may be going through. It takes two people to do the exercise, but it will be well worth the effort. See for yourself.

After enduring the "Spelling Bee" exercise, you will have some idea of the discomfort and distress that many children experience every day. We exaggerated the spelling test conditions for you. However, common, everyday situations present exaggerated problems for the children we are describing.

These children need a great deal of space for efficient writing; therefore, standard sizes of paper seem too small for their needs.

The Spelling Bee

To better understand the discomfort that many children feel when they are required to sit straight and still, imagine yourself in a typical classroom on a Friday morning, almost religiously preparing for the universal weekly spelling test. You will need someone who can play "teacher" for you for a few minutes, and you will need a pencil and a small piece of paper (about 2 inches by 3 inches). Sit in a straight chair at a table and extend your legs straight out in front of you, keeping them raised off the floor. Don't brace or prop your legs on anything. Hold the pencil in the hand you do not normally use for writing. Now, keeping your legs raised in front of you, use your nondominant hand to write on the small piece of paper. Have the "teacher" dictate the following words to you at a rate of one word every second. Be certain that the "teacher" allows you no more than one second on each word:

elbow	doctor
sunshine	zebra
animal	transportation
Wednesday	mother
dinner	

How Did You Do?

Did you finish all the words? Did you keep up? Are the words legible? Are you proud of the way your paper looks? Would you want this paper displayed on the bulletin board? Do you think that this paper adequately reflects your intelligence? Would you like a penmanship grade on this paper? Are your legs still raised as they are supposed to be? Would you like to go through school all day sitting and writing like this? Are you comfortable?

Their motor coordination is generally so poor that their writing is as labored as yours was with your nondominant hand. They are at least as uncomfortable in the "normal" sitting position as you were with your legs extended in front of you. (If you weren't too uncomfortable after several seconds, try sitting that way for several hours, as children are expected to do in school. Now you know why some children call school "torture.")

They need considerably more time for average writing tasks, so the normal amount of writing time seems very short to them. While most teachers would not dictate spelling words at a rate of one every second, the length of time typically allowed for a task is really too short for the child who is uncomfortable.

The Source of Discomfort

What causes this discomfort and the inefficiency that arises from it? Is it lack of effort by the child? Is it poor discipline by the parents, the teachers, or both? Is it that the child is "all boy" or "naturally active?" Is it ADHD? A major reason why these children can't sit still is *none of the above.*

These children can't sit still because they are extremely uncomfortable in "normal" sitting positions. They are uncomfortable because a reflex is pulling their bodies in two different directions. This reflex makes it as difficult for children to do their schoolwork as it was for you to complete the spelling test in the "Spelling Bee" exercise.

In this book we will tell you what this reflex is, what it does to your children, and what you can do about it.

2. The Symmetric Tonic Neck Reflex

Just what is this reflex that makes some children so uncomfortable by pulling their bodies in two different directions? Knowing what the reflex is will help you to understand better how it may affect your children. The cure for the problem will make more sense if you understand the cause of the problem. To explain that cause, we will first review the early stages of child development.

Early Childhood Development

In the beginning, all essential movements made by the newborn child are actually reflexes. Motor development occurs as children gain con-

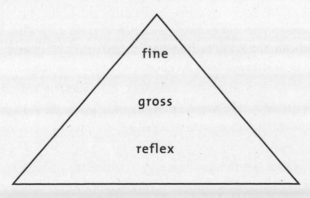

FIGURE 2.1. **The Three Levels of Coordination**

Some Early Reflexes

Reflexes are automatic responses to specific stimulation from the surroundings. (Anselmo and Franz 1995) The symmetric tonic neck reflex is one of the reflexes present in infants. The following table describes some of the many other newborn reflexes.

Infant Reflexes

Reflex	Appears	Disappears	Description
Rooting	Newborn	Six months	Infant turns toward a gentle touch of the cheek around the infant's mouth.
Sucking	Newborn	Six months	Infant sucks on objects placed in the infant's mouth.
Babinski	Newborn	Six months	Toes of the foot spread when the sole of the foot is gently stroked.
Grasping	Newborn	Six months	Infant firmly grasps an object when the palm of the hand is gently stroked.

trol over the movement of their bodies. Children aren't born coordinated; coordination develops through three basic levels (see figure 2.1):

1. reflex-motor (automatic movement, e.g., sucking reflex)
2. gross-motor (large muscle movement, e.g., throwing a ball)
3. fine-motor (small muscle movement, e.g., writing, coloring)

The reflex level provides the basis, or foundation, for all motor development. Reflex development comes first, followed in order by gross motor development and then fine motor development.

Reflex	Appears	Disappears	Description
Moro (startle)	Newborn	Six months	Infant extends arms and legs and then pulls them back to the body in a hugging motion in response to a quick falling backward of the infant's head or a loud disruption.
Protective reactions	Newborn	Six months	Infant moves head from side to side to dislodge a blanket covering the infant's face.
Blinking	Newborn	Permanent	Infant blinks eyes when an object comes too near.
Coughing	Newborn	Permanent	Infant coughs in response to various stimuli irritating the throat.
Sneezing	Newborn	Permanent	Infant sneezes in response to various stimuli irritating the nasal passages.
Gag	Newborn	Permanent	Infant gags in response to blockage of the throat.

These levels build on each other. If any one of these levels is not properly developed, there will be some trouble in the development of the level or levels above it. *Proper reflex development,* therefore, is basic and necessary to complete motor development. It is important to remember that a reflex is an automatic reaction—an involuntary action—and action that controls the movement of the body. (An example is the blinking reflex for protection of the eye. For a list of reflexes, see "Some Early Reflexes" on page 16.) The particular reflex we are concerned with here is the Symmetric Tonic Neck Reflex.

Dr. Miriam Bender provided an explanation of how infants, initially controlled largely by reflexes, gradually override many of these reflexes:

The newborn infant is essentially a reflex organism. He survives because he roots, sucks, swallows, breathes, cries, coughs, sneezes, and eliminates body wastes reflexly. He moves his arms, legs, and head in reflex response to stimuli from his environment as well as in response to stimuli generated within his own body.

Each time the infant responds reflexly by movement, feedback from his movement and his body position reaches his brain by way of his proprioceptive system. This sensory system provides a continuous flow of information about the movements and positions of his body and its parts in relation to gravity. . . .

As the infant continues to integrate primitive reflex patterns and to recombine their parts into voluntary movements and patterns of coordinated movement, he begins to override and suppress the more primitive of these reflexes. . . . Now most of their movements, especially those of the arms and hands, are under increasing voluntary control. Only his patterns of early locomotion are still subject to reflex modification. . . .

In many ways, the process of developmental learning is like climbing a ladder. From a firm base of support, the climber's body spans the space of several rungs as he reaches up to grasp the highest one within easy reach. Once his grasp on this higher rung is firm, the climber is free to move his feet upward. . . .

So it is with learning. As the child achieves some skill in a more efficient method of information processing, he is free to abandon his least efficient method. (Bender 1976, p. 12)

The Role of the Symmetric Tonic Neck Reflex

The Symmetric Tonic Neck Reflex is an automatic movement that makes the top half of the body work in opposition to the bottom half: when the top half is straight, the bottom half bends, and vice versa. The Symmetric Tonic Neck Reflex (STNR) is so named because it is an automatic movement (a reflex) that makes the right and left sides of the body work together (symmetric). The reflex is activated by a change in the position of the neck (neck), which produces a change in the muscular tension (tonic). In other words, we are discussing and describing the

Symmetric: both sides of the body working together

Tonic: producing a change in muscular tension, or tone

Neck: activated by a change in the position of the neck

Reflex: an automatic action

From this point on, we will refer to this reflex as the STNR. The STNR is an automatic movement that affects both sides of the body. The STNR is not active at birth, but it develops when a baby is between four and eight months old. At that point, the STNR gains control over some of the child's motions.

Consider a baby who is six months old. Generally, babies at this age have good control of their heads. They have been able to raise their heads and look around for some time. However, when the STNR develops, the three body units—neck, arms, and legs—*automatically interact*. These three parts become essentially "tied together" by the reflex, so that movement of any *one* of these three body parts (neck, arms, or legs) automatically produces some movement in the other two parts. This is important and normal at this stage of the baby's development. Here is what happens:

1. The baby raises its head to look around.
   The reflex is activated by a change in the position of the neck.
2. The reflex causes the baby's arms to automatically straighten, lifting the chest from the floor.
3. The reflex causes the knees and hips to bend and pull the baby back onto its heels.

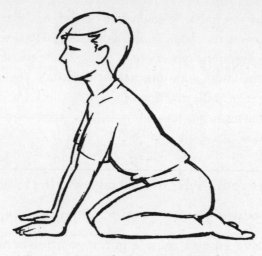

FIGURE 2.2. **The Cat Sit Position**

We call the resulting position the "cat sit" because the baby's position resembles that of a cat, sitting back on its haunches (see figure 2.2). It is as if the baby were divided in half at the waist: when the top half (that is, the arms and the neck) is straight, the bottom half (the legs) bends. In the figure, the child's neck and arms are straight while its legs are bent. When the bottom half straightens, the top half automatically bends. Once more for emphasis—the important fact to remember is the division of the body at the waist:

NECK ⎫ neck and arms work together
ARMS ⎬
—————
LEGS   legs work opposite from the neck and arms

When the STNR is in control, the bottom half of the body automatically does the opposite of whatever the top half of the body does. At this stage of development, the action of the STNR is normal and important. Its purpose is to pull the baby up off of its stomach into the cat sit position in preparation for crawling. Once in the cat sit position, the baby begins to rock back and forth.

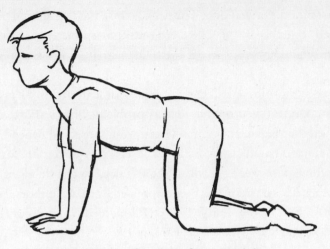

FIGURE 2.3. **The Crawling Position**

Eventually, during this rocking stage, one hand moves out farther, then the other, and the body moves from the cat sit into the crawling position (see figure 2.3), and the child begins to crawl.*

At this stage of development, the STNR is in control of the baby's body. Through the process of normal motor development—rocking and crawling—the child's body is controlled less and less by the STNR.

The Importance of Crawling to the Maturation of the STNR

By two years of age, if the child has crawled *enough*—at least six months—and *properly,* the child should be in control of its body, rather than having the STNR in control (Milani-Comparetti and Gidoni 1967). This six months of crawling can be achieved through the combination of the crawling months plus the intermittent crawling done in

---

* Technically speaking, *creeping* is the term given to a child's position with hands and knees on the floor, stomach off the floor. However, the term *crawling* is more popularly used to describe that position. For the purposes of this book, we have chosen to use the more popular term, *crawling*.

the first months of walking. The neck, arms, and legs should no longer be "tied" together by the reflex. No one knows exactly how this comes about. What happens, then, if the reflex activity is *not* suppressed?

> Most authorities agree that children with learning problems have some kind of neurophysiological problem. Piaget (1952) maintained that higher functional levels presuppose and depend upon the functional efficiency of lower levels. Any deficit and/or malfunction at a lower level will affect all related higher levels of functioning. This position has been expressed by many authors: Frostig (1966), Flax (1968), Early (1969), Dillon, Heath and Biggs (1970), and Kephart (1971). (O'Dell 1973, p. 19)

Dr. Miriam Bender explained the vital role performed by crawling:

> The coordinated movements of creeping promote better differentiation of movement. This ability to move one part of the body independently but in synchrony with other body parts is essential to flexible and efficient use of the body. . . .
>
> [Some] children creep so poorly or find the attempt so frustrating that they seek early escape into walking. These children, and those who do not progress to creeping in play, lack the motor experiences necessary to achieve suppression of the Symmetric TNR; and some degree of active reflex response lingers on. As long as a reflex remains active enough for its response to modify a child's voluntary movements, it will interfere with optimal development. (Bender 1976, p. 22)

In the proper crawling posture, the baby is crawling forward on hands and knees, with the head up and the stomach off the floor. The importance of the cat sit and crawling positions to proper crawling can be seen from B. L. White's description of a child's progression to crawling:

> Anna gets herself up on all fours in a crawling position and rocks back and forth as if she has an idea but cannot quite implement it.

Her first crawling movements are backward, but she gradually learns to move forward. Movements enhance new motor skills and satisfy curiosity, which encourages Anna to conduct first-hand investigation of her environment. (White 1990)

"Cross lateral movements, like a baby's crawling . . . activate both hemispheres [of the brain] in a balanced way . . . Cognitive function is heightened and ease of learning increases." (Hannaford 1995, p. 81)

A baby should crawl in the proper posture for at least six months to allow sufficient time for the STNR to be suppressed, as Dr. Miriam Bender has described:

An active symmetric TNR is essential if the child is to conquer gravity and rise first to his hands and knees and then to standing. It is equally essential, however, that he suppress the reflex response once he has learned to achieve these positions voluntarily, if he is to progress to efficient locomotion by creeping and later by walking.

The infant begins this process of suppression by "rocking." Once the infant finds himself on hands and knees in the reflex-evoked position, he begins trying to move about in that position. But when the infant pushes forward from his knees, the reflex asserts itself in reverse and he finds himself flat on the floor again.

So—the child begins rocking forward and back, forward and back, experimenting with the movement and exploring his own capabilities. Gradually he increases his voluntary control and achieves a smooth reciprocal creeping gait.

Creeping is . . . the most productive of important learning experiences. Efficient creeping, as a result of its rhythmic alternating pattern of movement, requires differentiated and synchronized control of limbs and head. As the child creeps, the proprioceptive information he receives from his movements is consistent and repeated over and over with minimal variation.

The coordinated movements of creeping promote better differentiation of movement. This ability to move one part of the body independently but in synchrony with other body parts is essential. (Bender 1976, pp. 20–22)

When a child gains independent control of his or her neck, arms, and legs, we say that the STNR is "mature." This maturing of the STNR is achieved through proper and enough (at least six months) crawling. (See "Alternative Forms of Locomotion That Do Not Mature the STNR" on page 31.) You must *not* try to force a baby to crawl. Rather, you should encourage crawling and provide ample opportunity for crawling. Fortunately, most babies begin to crawl between five and eight months of age and begin to walk at about one year of age. "We have known for years that children who miss the vitally important crawling stage may exhibit learning difficulties later on." (Hannaford 1995, p. 100) This book is about babies *who do not crawl at all, who crawl for a very short time, who do not crawl in the proper fashion, who walk early, or who are in playpens, braces, walkers, baby swings/bouncers, or other crawling inhibitors for long periods of time.*

How to Enhance the Normal Development of an STNR in a Baby

Do's . . .

- Do place babies on their stomachs frequently when they are awake. Be certain to monitor them.
- Do encourage crawling.
- Do allow ample opportunity for crawling.

Do Not's . . .

- Do not put babies in walkers, bouncers, etc.
- Do not overdo the use of playpens.
- Do not encourage early walking (before one year of age).

Reasons for Not Crawling Long Enough and Properly: Genetic and Environmental

A strong STNR (an STNR that remains in control of the child's movements beyond the age when it would ordinarily have matured and disappeared) may be genetically caused. We inherit eye color, bone structure, and our reflexes; the tendency toward a strong STNR may also be inherited. We often see many of the same problems in more than one family member.

On the other hand, the cause could be environmental—occurring in situations that are well-intentioned, or unavoidable, or inadvertent, but nevertheless interfering with the crawling process. Many babies who could crawl long enough and properly *lose the opportunity* to crawl because they spend too much time in playpens, bouncers, swings, walkers, etc. Playpens can occasionally be put to good use for safety purposes, but time spent in such a confined area should be limited. (The best use we ever heard for a playpen was by a mother of five children under the age of seven. She would get into the playpen to read the newspaper while her babies slept or played nearby.)

Walkers, on the other hand, we would like to see banned from the face of the earth. They deny the child the opportunity to crawl at all. Many professionals have recommended the banning of walkers for reasons of lack of safety and interference with child development. Recently, some of the safety hazards of walkers have been addressed by the creation of new design requirements set by government guidelines. But new product designs cannot address the developmental interference caused by walkers. Research indicates that the use of walkers not only prohibits crawling, but, contrary to popular belief, actually delays the development of independent walking. Do not be fooled by the charming new stand-up-behind-and-push toys. They are simply the twenty-first century's version of baby walkers. A baby cannot crawl in a walker.

Some babies are too ill in their early lives to be placed on the floor for crawling. Some babies are carried too much, and their fat, little baby knees never touch the floor. Some babies have casts or braces on their legs or arms, which will, unfortunately, interfere with crawling. Some babies are kept off the floor because of drafty, cold, or rough floors. Some babies are in homes with very little space available for crawling. Many babies, recently, because of the "Back to Sleep" movement, are never even placed on their stomachs to be able to crawl.

A Consequence of the "Back to Sleep" Movement: Not Crawling Long Enough and Not Properly

Since 1992, when the American Academy of Pediatrics made a formal recommendation that *healthy* infants be placed on their backs to sleep (supine position), there has been a movement to have infants and babies sleep on their backs as much as possible to avoid the danger of sudden infant death syndrome (SIDS). That recommendation has been embraced by physicians and parents around the world, with the gratifying result that the incidence of SIDS has decreased.

While the "Back to Sleep" movement has been successful in lowering the incidence of SIDS, current studies are bringing to light some unexpected negative side effects of having babies on their backs so much of the time. Probably because the benefit of the "Back to Sleep" movement (reduction of SIDS) far outweighs any negative side effects, the information of the negative side effects has, so far, received less attention. It is almost taboo to question a program that has been so wondrously effective in reducing infant death. However, it is fortunately possible and easily achievable to attain the beneficial effects of the "Back to Sleep" program while avoiding the negative side effects. Consequently, we can afford to address some of the potential difficulties brought about by the "Back to Sleep" movement.

Infants spending time primarily on their backs are slower to develop good head control and strong neck muscles. (Center for the Advancement of Health 2000) (Konishi 1987) This delay in development often causes a tilting of the head and shortened neck muscles—

twisted neck (torticollis). (McGee 2000) (Watson 2000) Reports indicate a dramatic increase in the incidence of flattened head (plagiocephaly) and twisted neck since so many babies are spending so much time on their backs. (Hagan 2003) (Pontius 2001)

Because babies are spending so much time on their backs when awake as well as when asleep, they are not developing the muscles and motor skills necessary to roll over. Nor are they comfortable on their stomachs on the less and less frequent occasions when they are *placed* on their stomachs. (Foundation for the Study of Infant Deaths 2000) "A baby on his or her back is neurologically upside down. It is not possible for a baby in this position to crawl or creep. Consequently, organization of the sub-cortical brain areas cannot occur." (Loyd 2000)

There is consensus among researchers, developmental specialists, and pediatricians that they ". . . are seeing increasing numbers of babies who never crawl at all . . ." (*New York Times* 2001) "The 'Back to Sleep' campaign has spawned another unanticipated result, Aponte [chairman of the departments of pediatrics and ambulatory care at North General Hospital in New York City] says. Children seem to be bypassing the crawling stage." (Gardner 2003)

Sadly, some of these researchers/specialists are convincing themselves that skipping the crawling stage is an acceptable side effect of the life-saving results of the "Back to Sleep" program. (*Indianapolis Star* 2001) Some have gone so far as to say that crawling is no longer considered a developmental milestone. (Porretto 2003) It would appear that these professionals, in their zeal to encourage the continuation of putting babies on their backs to sleep to prevent SIDS, are willing to sacrifice the major developmental milestone of crawling. It is, however, neither necessary nor acceptable to diminish the importance of crawling in order to obtain the best results from the "Back to Sleep" campaign.

There are even some who are saying that crawling is not necessary so long as normal development occurs. But how in the world can normal development occur if a baby skips the important milestone of crawling? "While it is true that these babies appear to develop normally as they learn to walk and talk, they have not had an opportunity to finish important sub-cortical development." (Loyd 2000)

From the beginning of the awareness of developmental stages, crawling has always been listed as a major milestone (Executive Parent 2003) (Kinderstart 2000)—and for good reasons.

According to many authorities, crawling is essential to

- " . . . organize sub-cortical, non-thinking areas of the central nervous system.
- . . . form the foundation upon which all future learning and development is constructed.
- [prevent] . . . random, confused, and disorganized learning. . . ." (Loyd 2000)
- develop neurological organization.
- facilitate visual tracking. (Gilbert 2001)
- coordinate the development of both sides of the brain.
- develop sensory and motor systems and general motor skills. (Fysh 2003)
- develop shoulders, wrists, and small muscles of the hands.
- begin bilateral coordination. (Loikith 2001)
- MATURE THE SYMMETRIC TONIC NECK REFLEX.

There is an obviously simple solution to the problems arising from having babies on their backs too much: *Put them on their stomachs when they are awake and can be monitored.* Implementing this "Tummy to Play" recommendation will give babies many more opportunities for neck and upper torso development, neurological and sub-cortical organization, and the development of visual tracking and the basic motor skills that lead to crawling.

Fortunately, the American Academy of Pediatrics Task Force on Infant Positioning and SIDS has modified the original recommendation to include "tummy time" while the infant is awake and observed. This time spent on the stomach is being recommended for developmental reasons and to help prevent flattened heads. Unfortunately, the "Tummy to Play" recommendation is not receiving the same emphasis as the "Back to Sleep" campaign, probably because the issues are not so serious. (However, it appears that at least the toy manufacturers are alert to the "Tummy to Play" recommendation. Recently there has been a considerable increase in the design and production of toys that promote "tummy time.")

Missing out on "tummy time" may not be life threatening. Nevertheless, spending most of the waking and sleeping hours on the back can create havoc in the child's development, significantly and negatively affecting future comfort and achievement. The "Back to Sleep" campaign has been blessedly effective in reducing SIDS. However, we urge you not to allow those who promote the valuable "Back to Sleep" campaign to arbitrarily eliminate the important developmental milestone of crawling in order to justify a negative outcome they had not anticipated—not crawling long enough and properly.

We can have the best of both worlds: "Back to Sleep" and "Tummy to Play."

The Consequences of Not Crawling Long Enough and Properly

Crawling has long been recognized as an important aspect of child development. Babies should crawl properly and extensively for about six months or longer (from approximately six months of age to twelve months of age). But with the advent of inhibitors to crawling (e.g., walkers, bouncers, playpens, etc.), in addition to lack of time on their stomachs, today's babies in increasing numbers are missing out on the important developmental milestone of crawling. This lack of crawling is producing devastating effects.

Relationship to Sense of Direction (Directionality)

The development of directionality begins with a child's crawling in infancy. As children crawl, they gain an internal awareness of the two sides of their bodies. This awareness of "sidedness," or laterality, eventually develops into a sense of direction. Directionality is the awareness of our own right- and left-sidedness in the world around us. While a child may turn right or left in a walker, the use of both arms and both legs in crawling provides a significantly greater proprioceptive feedback* to the infant. This feedback helps to establish laterality.

Children who do not crawl at all, or who crawl for a very short period of time, or who walk very early, or who crawl "funny" will miss out on this essential stage in the development of directionality. These children are usually delayed in learning right from left. This directional confusion often extends into reversals of letters and numbers. They frequently resort to external clues to help with right-or-left identification, such as which hand has a mole, a wart, a wristwatch, or some other identifying mark. Although this external system of right-or-left identification is helpful, it is slower and less efficient than the quicker internal awareness that begins with the crawling process.

Relationship to Intelligence

We have found that there is no connection or correlation between the maturation of the STNR (for which proper and sufficient crawling is necessary) and the child's level of intelligence. While early walking may be a sign of superior intelligence, it may also be an indication of a very strong STNR. It may indicate both. *The maturation of the STNR is dependent upon proper and enough crawling (at least six months), not on the child's level of intelligence.* However, an immature STNR can make a child appear less intelligent by interfering with the child's learning and performance.

Relationship to the STNR

If, for any reason, a baby does not crawl long enough (at least six months) and properly, the STNR will continue to control the baby's body. In other words, the top half of the body will want to be straight when the bottom half bends, and vice versa.

If at this point you are feeling guilty about having your baby in a

---

* Proprioceptive feedback is the sensation from active muscles and joints that supplies information about limb position and movement of parts of the body, monitored and utilized by the individual for production of more accurate responses.

Alternative Forms of Locomotion That Do Not Mature the STNR

There are many common forms of locomotion for babies besides crawling. These include:

- scooting on their bottoms
- rolling across the floor
- pulling themselves forward on their forearms, dragging their legs, in what we call an "army crawl"
- crawling with hands and feet on the floor, with their bottoms in the air, in what we all a "camel walk"
- hitching forward, dragging one leg
- hopping like a frog or rabbit
- "swimming" across the floor on their stomachs
- crawling primarily backward
- walking early

Unfortunately, these forms of movement do not mature the STNR, and the reflex stays in control.

playpen or walker, or about encouraging early walking, take thirty seconds to feel guilty—and then forget it! You were trying to be a good parent, and you are just now finding out about the STNR.

Most babies, fortunately, crawl properly and enough, but at least 10 percent do not. This percentage is derived from the well-known statistic that 10 to 20 percent of the general population is learning disabled (Lerner 1997). In a groundbreaking study by Miriam Bender, Dr. Bender found that at least 75 percent of that learning-disabled population has an immature STNR contributing to their learning disabilities (Bender 1971). This translates into at least 25 million people in the United States—children and adults—who still have not matured the STNR. We are talking about *at least* two or three children in every regular classroom who have not matured the STNR. We are not saying that all learning-disabled children have an immature STNR, nor that an immature STNR is the only cause of learning disorders. We are saying that at least 75 percent of children with learning difficulties have an immature STNR as a main contributing factor.

Remember:

- A baby must crawl properly and enough (at least six months) to mature the STNR.
- The STNR should mature by the age of two.
- If a baby does not crawl properly and enough (at least six months) an immature STNR remains in control of the baby's body.
- If a child has not matured the STNR by the age of two, the child will not just outgrow the effects of the immature STNR without special help.

Now you know what the STNR is, how it is supposed to mature, and how often it does not mature. This book is about children and adults who are frequently diagnosed as ADHD. What most of them may really have is an immature STNR.

Read on to discover how an immature STNR creates extreme physical and/or psychological distress for children when they are required to sit still for extended periods.

3. Looking for Clues to the Real Problem

Because of the frustration, aggression, and inflexibility that STNR children often display, many of them are misdiagnosed as having primary emotional problems that are causing their academic and behavioral difficulties. We are convinced that it is usually the other way around! Academic failure causes the emotional distress. Because of an immature STNR, most of these children fail to meet academic and behavioral demands. In many cases, the academic and behavioral problems are primary; the emotional problems are secondary, an emotional overlay.

Many of the children we see at our clinic have previously been taken to child psychologists, psychiatrists, and guidance clinics for help with emotional, behavioral, or academic problems. The following comments from some of these professionals are frequently reported to us by parents:

"He's just all boy."
"He's just immature."
"She'll outgrow it."
"You're too permissive," or the other side of that coin,
"You're too strict."
"You're an overly protective mother."
"You're too demanding a father."
"She needs to try a little harder."

"He's just not interested in school."

"He's lazy."

"He's just clumsy; learn to live with it."

"He's just not interested in that subject."

"He needs to be on medication."

We strongly disagree with most of these comments and diagnoses. We agree that, upon occasion, children's basic problems might be caused by either overly protective or overly permissive parents. Also, upon occasion, children might appear to coast in their schoolwork, seeming to put forth minimal effort. We emphatically disagree with the attitude that these children are lazy or that children must resign themselves to being awkward. We are sick of hearing that these children are just immature and that they'll outgrow their problems, or that medication will correct all these problems. We strongly believe that an immature STNR is often the root cause of chronic academic and behavioral problems.

Medical (Mis)Diagnosis and (Mis)Treatment

In our society, parents typically take their children to the family doctor for all types of problems—academic and behavioral problems included. Although physicians are not trained to deal with academic problems, they often give advice in educational matters, an area outside their expertise. (Physicians tend to become very upset when people not trained in medicine give medical advice. We wish they would practice what they preach.)

Because STNR children are usually in the examining room with the doctor for no more than five to ten minutes, STNR children generally do not display their overly active behavior to the physician in that short period of time. Physicians would be well-advised to consult with their receptionists to obtain a more accurate picture of the children's activity level over an extended period of time. Often, when the mother requests help for her overly active child, the physician will, as a result of limited observation of the child's behavior, misdiagnose the child's overactivity as being a problem of the mother or the teacher or both, rather than a problem of the child.

Some physicians will frequently diagnose the STNR child to be a normal, active, "all boy" type who will outgrow any minor problems if "the women in his life will just get off his back." This misdiagnosis is certainly unfair to the mothers and teachers, for they will feel guilty and frustrated. It is even more unfair to the children, however, for they will then receive no help at all for their STNR problems. Occasionally, these STNR children are misdirected to psychologists and psychiatrists who try to convince the family that the problems are primarily psychological. (We must note that the average physician is unaware of the behavioral and educational implications of the immature STNR. The STNR research has come through education, rather than through medicine, and the medical profession tends to disregard any research other than its own.)

Drug Therapy

Far too many physicians are too quick to diagnose the STNR child as ADHD (see "Diagnostic Criteria for Attention Deficit/ Hyperactivity Disorder" on page 36). The typical medical treatment for behavioral problems and hyperactivity is drug therapy. (Miller 1997, p. 80) Although medication can be beneficial in some cases, drug therapy attempts to treat the symptoms but doesn't even address the basic problem in STNR cases. If the behavioral problem is primarily caused by an immature STNR, maturing the reflex through our exercise program makes more sense than resorting to drug therapy. Drug therapy, with all its possible negative side effects, is frequently superficial, insufficient, and often totally ineffective in STNR cases. (See Appendix A, "To Drug or Not to Drug.")

Drug therapy will not mature an immature STNR.

Placing Blame

Not only do many physicians deal ineffectively with children's academic and behavioral problems, but many educators are also guilty of resisting new information and alternative methods. It has been

Diagnostic Criteria for Attention-Deficit/Hyperactivity Disorder

The following list of ADHD symptoms could just as easily describe children with an immature STNR. We strongly recommend the consideration of remediating for an immature STNR before embarking on the traditional drug therapy.

- Frequently fails to pay attention to details/makes careless mistakes
- Frequently has trouble maintaining attention in school or at play
- Frequently does not appear to listen when spoken to directly
- Frequently does not follow through on directions and fails to complete homework or duties at work
- Frequently has difficulty organizing tasks and activities
- Frequently avoids, seems to dislike, or seems reluctant to attempt activities that require sustained mental effort
- Frequently loses things necessary for tasks or activities
- Frequently is easily distracted by extraneous stimuli
- Frequently is forgetful in daily activities
- Frequently fidgets or squirms in chair
- Frequently leaves seat in classroom or in situations where remaining seated is expected
- Frequently runs about or climbs excessively in situations in which it is inappropriate
- Frequently has difficulty playing quietly
- Frequently seems "driven by a motor"
- Frequently talks excessively
- Frequently blurts out answers before questions have been completed
- Frequently has difficulty awaiting turn
- Frequently interrupts in conversations or games

Source: *DSM-IV-TR* American Psychiatric Association, © 2000.

our experience that many administrators and teachers frequently cling to traditional (mis)interpretations of academic and behavioral difficulties. These so-called explanations range from blaming the children totally to blaming the parents totally to blaming the children and the parents. Unfortunately, even after we have explained how the immature STNR causes many of these problems, some administrators and teachers still seem to have to *blame* somebody. They reject the STNR explanation, not because the explanation does not make sense, but because they seem to have a need for someone to be at fault.

"Many of the children who have learning problems have this lack of coordination. They have the same faulty neurological organization. With a child like that, the parent can't win. If he refuses to pressure the child into doing more of what he cannot do at school, he is accused of not caring; and if he does, he just might make matters worse. It is not a matter of the parent not caring—it is a question of not knowing how to fix the problem.

"The teacher, too, has a problem. She is accused by the parents of not teaching the child properly." (Gold 1997, p. 154)

Parents blame children and teachers.
Teachers blame children and parents.

Notice who is "caught" in the middle. Children "get it" from both sides.

Blaming someone will not mature an immature STNR.

Increased Discipline
More fault-finding, disguised as constructive criticism, comes from relatives and friends:

"You're not teaching our grandchildren any discipline."
"Why don't you teach your kids some table manners?"
"Why is Johnny jumping up from the table all the time?"

This outside criticism increases the frustrations and pressures that are already burdening the parents. The parents, in turn, bear down on the children. This extra discipline rarely improves their behavior and usually serves only to increase the frustration and pressures that are already burdening the children. Many parents, literally in tears, have told us, "Other people just don't know what it's like. No matter how much we discipline him [or her], it doesn't seem to do any good."

We can assure you that these STNR children have been disciplined—grounded, denied privileges, spanked, sent to their rooms, yelled at—more than relatives and friends would ever believe. This extra discipline is an attempt to treat symptoms, but it does not even address the basic problem.

Extra discipline will not mature an immature STNR.

Behavior Modification

When it becomes obvious that extra discipline will not get the job done, the "modern" approach is often to try behavior modification. Behavior modification is a very carefully planned use of rewards and punishments for eliminating undesirable behavior or establishing desirable behavior or both. (This is a rather simplistic definition, but it will serve the purpose here.)

Behavior modification can definitely help to establish certain behaviors that are within an individual's abilities. Many STNR children have been subjected to behavior modification programs designed to keep them in their seats. Some of these programs give the appearance of moderate success at first, but, in time, the STNR children develop other tension-releasing or disruptive behaviors. Many behavior modification programs fail completely because they make demands beyond the STNR child's abilities.

Remember that STNR children *cannot* sit still *comfortably* and pay attention easily. Even though behavior modification may be somewhat successful in helping children sit in their seats, it *cannot* help them to sit in their seats *comfortably* and pay attention easily. Even though behavior modification may be somewhat successful in helping children to begin their writing assignments, it *cannot* help them write *easily*.

Behavior modification will not mature an immature STNR.

STNR Children in Favorite Positions—Postural Clues

Early on, the interference of an immature STNR may not be noticed. Young children usually are allowed a great deal of postural freedom, flexibility, and mobility, so the child with an immature STNR is frequently able to find a comfortable position. Children in kindergarten and first grade are frequently allowed to lie on the floor, walk around the room, or stand to do their work, and they are not ordinarily kept at any one task for a long period of time, so the child with an immature STNR is usually able to escape the discomfort that the reflex causes. However, when a child is required to stay in the socially approved sitting position, the reflex immaturity causes problems.

Picture the position of a student's body in the "appropriate" sitting position: the knees and hips are bent, and the feet are flat on the floor—the child is *sitting up straight!* Everyone loves to see it! However, if the child's body is controlled by an immature STNR, even only partially, he or she would be far more comfortable, when sitting with the knees and hips bent, if the arms were straight. When the child's legs are bent, the arms would "prefer" to be straight, and vice-versa.

Remember: When the STNR is still in control (immature), the upper part of the body is more comfortable doing the opposite of what the lower part does, and the lower part is more comfortable doing the opposite of what the upper part does. If the neck and arms are bent, the legs are more comfortable straight; if the legs are bent (as when sitting), the arms would be more comfortable straight.

If the STNR caused children's arms to actually shoot straight out in front of them when their legs were bent, most teachers and parents would realize at once that these children had a problem of some kind, though a few might never notice. However, the reflex interference is not that obvious. We are essentially talking about normal children who are still somewhat, but not totally, under the control of the reflex. These children may be able to sit normally and may be able to sit still, but *they cannot sit comfortably,* and *they cannot sit still for long periods of time.*

Many of these children are not aware that they are more uncomfortable than the children around them. They have no frame of reference except the way their own bodies feel. The situation is rather like that of the child who has poor distance vision and, therefore, supposes that everyone has trouble seeing what is written on the chalkboard.

Some children with an immature STNR *are* aware of their discomfort and come to despise any task that requires sitting. Some, however, may think that something must be wrong with *them,* since they cannot sit still like the rest of their classmates. Often they begin a series of movements aimed at relieving the physical tension they are feeling when required to sit. In the effort to make themselves comfortable, they frequently try to assume positions in which half of the body can be bent while the other half is straight. Often they give up on comfort and just try to "lock" their bodies into their chairs, thereby meeting the demand for an acceptable sitting position.

We are not being critical of teachers in general. Most teachers work really hard to help children learn. Most teachers do not know about the educational effects of an immature STNR. However, numerous telltale signs and clues indicate an immature STNR in children and adults. Many of these signs are readily observable in the way individuals sit (or don't sit).

The Reachers

If STNR children are required to sit up, with their legs bent and their feet flat on the floor, their arms are more comfortable straight; therefore, these children may reach forward across their desks, attempting to write with their arms extended. (See figure 3.1.) They sometimes manage to extend their arms by gripping the back of the chair in front of them, much to the annoyance of the child sitting in that chair.

A boy named Joshua introduced us to another solution to the discomfort of sitting conventionally.

Joshua was an eight-year-old boy whose parents brought him to see us because of a basic coordination problem. Among other symptoms they described, they mentioned that he had "booming" headaches at the end of every school day. Fearing a brain tumor,

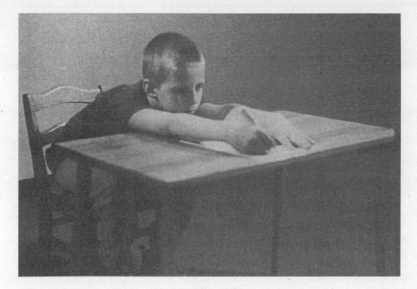

FIGURE 3.1. **The Reaching Position**

the parents had taken Joshua to two neurologists, who found nothing wrong neurologically. Then, thinking that the headaches might be caused by an eye problem, they took him to an optometrist and an ophthalmologist; neither found anything wrong.

During our interview of Joshua, he said that he had a great deal of writing to do in school. His teacher, Joshua said, was " . . . real big on having us stay in our seats." Joshua's hand hurt when he wrote for an extended period, but he had found a way to keep his hand from hurting. To avoid discomfort in his arm and hand, yet stay in his seat as his teacher required, Joshua had devised his own method of writing. He put his paper on the floor by his foot and leaned over to write, with his arms extended straight down and his head hanging nearly upside down.

We suggested to his parents the possibility that his headaches might be the result of having his head hanging down much of the day. Surely no child would *choose* to write in such a position unless it was more comfortable in some way. His teacher was trying to be flexible by allowing Joshua to take an unusual position as long as he did his work and stayed in his seat. She did not associate his headaches with his writing position. Not all headaches are caused by an immature STNR, of course, but Joshua's headaches were. When we matured his STNR, and he no longer had to hang upside down to do his written work, his headaches disappeared.

Most teachers would probably not allow children to put their papers on the floor as Joshua did and hang upside down to write. Teachers generally require children to put their papers on their desks and to sit up straight while they write. (Remember that teachers are also just now finding out about the STNR.)

And so these children assume another position, trying to get comfortable.

The Slouchers

If STNR children are seated at a desk or table and bend their necks and arms in the usual writing position, their legs are more comfortable extended straight out in front of them (see figure 3.2). We see children (especially older children, whose legs are long enough) sliding down in their seats, stretching their legs out into the aisles, creating a potential hazard. A variation of this posture involves the children bracing their extended legs on the chairs in front of them. While this is more comfortable for the STNR children, it is frequently very annoying to the children in front of them.

You can begin to see how these children can be inadvertently distracting to their neighbors (and even to themselves). This slouching position tends to make them appear lazy, uninterested in what is being taught in class, and even insolent. The teacher usually tells these children to "Sit up straight!" That is the first commandment of the classroom . . . well, maybe the second; the first is "Sit down."

And so these children assume another position, trying to get comfortable.

The Chair Tippers

If STNR children are tall enough (as older children usually are), they will attempt to straighten their legs by bracing their toes against

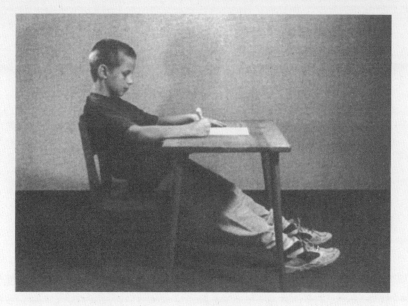

FIGURE 3.2. **The Slouching Position**

the floor and leaning back precariously, balancing on just the back legs of the chair. While this position may be more comfortable for the STNR children, it is certainly not safe and must not be allowed.

The Foot Lockers and Foot Sitters

If STNR children are not permitted to stretch their legs or arms, they will frequently "lock" their feet around the legs of the chair, especially when required to have their arms bent for writing or holding a book (see figure 3.3). What does this locking do for a child? The locking of the feet holds the legs still, helping the child to stay in the seat, as required. In a variation of this position, children sit on their feet. They may sit on one foot and then the other, or they may sit on both feet. However, frequently their feet "go to sleep" after a short period of time. Another postural change or shift is then required.

Remember: the upper and lower halves of the body do not want to be bent at the same time when under the influence of the immature STNR. Locking one half of the body helps keep it from moving. If the legs are not locked, there is usually considerable movement, squirming, and "antsiness." Because the three parts—neck, arms,

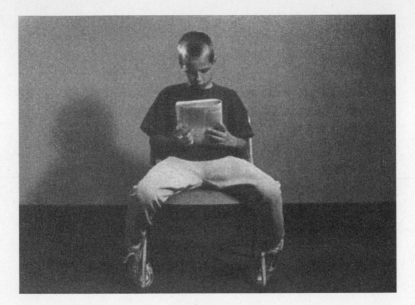

FIGURE 3.3. **The Foot Locking Position**

and legs—are still tied together by the immature STNR, when one part moves, or its position is even slightly changed, the immature STNR changes the muscular tension in the other two parts.

Think of the child who is copying material from the chalkboard. Every time the child looks up at the board or down at the paper, movements that require adjustments in the neck position, there is a change in the muscular tension in the arms and legs. As the child changes body positions, the pressure on the pencil changes, too. Frequently, the pencil point breaks because the child is unable to maintain consistent pressure on the pencil. STNR children make many trips to the pencil sharpener for this reason and also because going to the pencil sharpener is an acceptable excuse for getting up and moving around to relieve the discomfort that the child feels. Even if such children lock their legs and do not squirm, there is a continuous shifting and building-up of tension in their bodies, leading to fatigue and discomfort.

And so these children assume another position, trying to get comfortable.

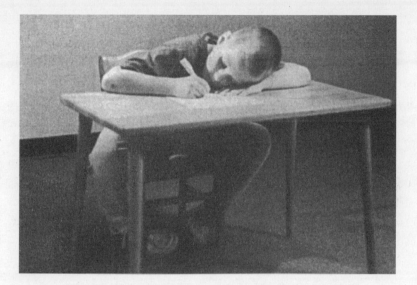

FIGURE 3.4. **The Head Resting Position**

The Head Resters

If STNR children lay their heads on their arms while writing, they sometimes manage to lock the upper half of their bodies in an immobile position, thereby controlling the STNR action (see figure 3.4). They may also hold their chins in the palms of their hands, resting their elbows on their desks, in an attempt to stabilize themselves. The more body parts they can lock or hold still, the better they can cope with the STNR. Some children can anchor their papers with their elbows in this position, while others seem unable to prevent twisting and skewing their papers as they write. Twisting and skewing, of course, do not generally contribute to the neatness of papers.

Teachers and parents are frequently appalled and disheartened by the appearance of the children's papers: smudged, sloppy, worn-through with erasures, crumpled, and just plain messy. STNR children are equally disheartened to see the pitiful results of so much time and effort and strain.

And so these children assume another position, trying to get comfortable.

The Standers

If STNR children are permitted to stand, they can comfortably bend their arms and necks while their legs are straight (see figure 3.5). Some STNR children will stand beside their desks, with one knee resting on the seat, attempting to be comfortable and at the same time to obey the teacher's rule, "Stay in your seat." Others may work their way to a counter or table or even to the teacher's desk, trying to find a suitable height for working while standing up.

One first-grade girl who was referred to our clinic by her teacher provided a vivid example of standing as a means of finding comfort. We call her case our Goldilocks story.

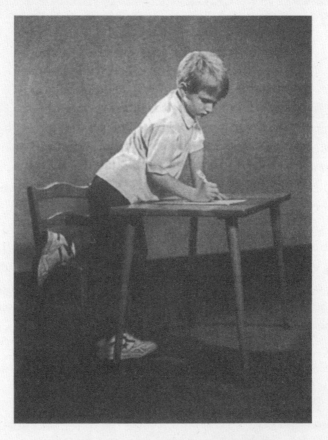

FIGURE 3.5. **The Standing Position**

Once upon a time, a teacher referred a first-grade girl to our clinic, suspecting an emotional problem. This little girl was at the teacher's elbow all day. The teacher didn't seem to be able to get out of the child's sight.

We visited the classroom frequently for several days of observation, and we soon discovered that the child was more interested in the teacher's desk than she was in the teacher. She didn't really need to be near the teacher; she needed the teacher's desk in order to write comfortably. Testing later determined that this child was bothered by an immature STNR. She wanted to *stand* to do her written work. Her first-grade desk was too low; the counter by the window was too high; but the teacher's desk was *juuust right*.

There certainly are instances of emotional problems in school-children. However, it has been our experience that many children who are thought to be emotionally disturbed are primarily suffering from an immature STNR. Unfortunately, they are often described as having primary behavioral or emotional problems.

And so these children assume another position, trying to get comfortable.

The Recliners

If STNR children lie on the floor, legs stretched out behind them, elbows bent, with their chins cupped in their hands, they are generally comfortable (see figure 3.6). (The upper body is bent, because the arms are bent at the elbows; the lower body is straight, because the legs are extended flat on the floor.) At home and in school during the earliest years, children are often allowed this position. They are comfortable, and, as a result, they may not squirm and fidget very much. Consequently, many parents are perplexed when told by teachers in higher grades that the same children do not sit still. Parents often respond, "He can lie on the floor and watch television by the hour without moving," never realizing that the child's reclining position improves comfort. Therefore, the child does not have to engage in the constant shifting, squirming search for comfort that the teacher sees in the classroom.

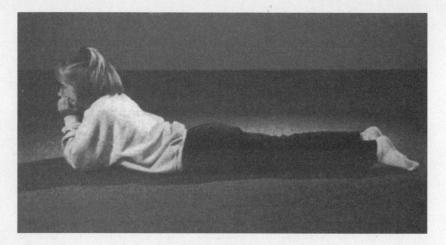

FIGURE 3.6. **The Reclining Position**

Some parents are annoyed when children lie on the floor or assume unusual positions to do homework rather than sitting at the kitchen table or at their newly purchased desks. One example of the conflict between a child's "creative posturing" and a parent's expectations was demonstrated by a boy named Larry, who usually studied spelling alone and then ran through a practice test with his father.

While Larry was studying the spelling words alone, he draped himself upside down on the sofa with his legs bent over the sofa's back, his body hanging over the front, and his head almost touching the floor. He put his arms straight up over his head, holding the spelling book. He seemed very content in this position.

Then Larry's father came in to dictate the spelling words. He insisted that his son sit at the table, "to be in a better position for studying." What the father missed, of course, was that Larry *had been studying.*

What Larry's *body* understood was that for him a "better position for studying" was not sitting at the table, but draped across the sofa. When sitting at the table with his father, Larry could maintain attention for only a very short time before beginning to fidget. Each study session began pleasantly but ended in an argument. The father was exasperated by his son's constant wiggling, and the son was frustrated by being so uncomfortable and still unable to please his father.

And so these children assume another position, trying to get comfortable.

The Squirmers

If STNR children are not allowed to assume any of the positions previously described, they just squirm all day, trying to make themselves comfortable in some position.

A second-grade boy named Billy was referred to us because of his learning problems. Along with some other difficulties, he had an immature STNR. His parents reported that Billy had begun walking very early, after crawling for no longer than several weeks. After hearing our description of the effects of the STNR, the parents agreed that, indeed, Billy seemed to be bothered by the reflex. STNR testing confirmed an immature reflex. (For a discussion of the STNR test, see "The STNR Test" on page 134.)

Billy was squirming to the point of being disruptive. His mother commented that even their family meals were disrupted because Billy was in constant motion. Dinner conversations were interrupted by "Sit down, Billy;" "Sit up straight, Billy;" "Billy, stop swinging your legs; you're kicking your sister;" and on and on. Dinner was not enjoyable for anyone in the family. The father said that Billy probably thought his name was "Billy Stop," because that was what he heard most of the time. These were very devoted and intelligent parents, and their comments to Billy were not angry or mean . . . just exasperated.

We suggested that they permit Billy to stand up at the dinner table to reduce his fidgeting. At first they were appalled. The teaching of manners was very important to them, and they didn't want Billy to think that he could stand up to eat whenever he wanted. We explained that sitting and eating were producing the same tension in Billy's arms and legs as sitting at a desk and writing. We assured them that allowing him to stand up to eat would be only a temporary measure, while we worked with Billy on a program to mature the STNR. They agreed to try it.

Billy's mother called about ten days later and said, "If nothing else comes from this program, we'll be happy. We've had our first pleasant meals in seven years."

A minor improvement? Hardly. One of the few times families are all together in today's society is at the dinner table. Here was a family that dreaded the dinner hour but was now able to enjoy it. Consider also the self-image Billy had been developing. Every time his name had been used at the dinner table, it was in a negative manner. He had begun to think he must be a very bad child, when in fact he was just very uncomfortable.

And so these children assume another position, and another and another, trying to get comfortable.

Body Language as a Postural Clue

A child's body language and the positions the child assumes in an attempt to get comfortable are powerful clues to the interference of the STNR. Do not be alarmed if you and your children occasionally assume some of these postures. Everyone will take these positions once in a while, but those who constantly avoid the socially accepted sitting position are giving postural clues to the discomfort caused by the immature STNR. While everybody assumes some of the positions occasionally, people with STNR immaturity assume these positions more frequently and persistently.

Clues to Look For
Behaviors can have many causes. However, the following behaviors are commonly caused by an immature STNR. If the child did not crawl properly or long enough, we can guarantee that there is

The STNR as a Factor in Learning Disabilities

Researchers at Emory University (Freides et al. 1980) concluded that:

> In . . . the symmetric tonic neck reflex, when the head tilts backward, the arms extend (stretch out) and the legs flex (bend), while the reverse occurs when the head tilts forward. If even partial components of this primitive organization are present, the ordinary business of looking up at the chalkboard and then down to the desk will play havoc with the muscle tone and movement of the arms and fingers. The child will display awkward movement, impaired attention, frustration, or withdrawal. . . . Systematic, controlled observations with stringent guards against observer bias confirmed causal evidence and prior less well-controlled studies that learning-disabled children are likely to suffer motor impairments. . . . Such relatively inconspicuous yet important defects are likely to exert an insidious influence, undermining attention, performance, and perhaps even self-concept.

Kenneth Dunn, of Queens College, and Rita Dunn, of St. John's University (Dunn and Dunn 1987), reported that "well-designed studies show that making youngsters sit upright in their seats does not necessarily make them more receptive to learning." They cited the following studies:

- Shea 1983, which identified students who performed significantly better while positioned "informally on cushions, pillows, couches, and carpeting";
- Hodges 1985, in which seventh- and eighth-graders obtained significantly higher mathematics scores when allowed postural flexibility;
- Della Valle 1984, which reported that 50 percent of a group of seventh-graders observed scored significantly higher when allowed to move around than when required to stay seated.

STNR interference. Be aware, though, that not all of the following behaviors have to be present to indicate STNR immaturity.

- Difficulty with sitting still in the "proper" position: stands up, fidgets, slouches, wraps feet around chair legs, sits on feet, lies down, changes position frequently.
- Difficulty with writing: writes laboriously, writes sloppily, writes very small or very large, breaks pencil points frequently, tries to stand up to write, avoids writing, loses place frequently when copying work from chalkboard or book.
- Difficulty with sense of direction: confuses left and right, needs extra time or a "marker" to determine left from right, reads and/ or writes "backward."
- Difficulty with coordination: tends to be clumsy or poorly coordinated; has trouble with skipping, marching, running and catching, running and throwing; avoids certain sports or certain positions in sports; prefers swimming underwater, or the breaststroke, or the butterfly stroke rather than freestyle.
- Difficulty with homework: avoids or postpones the beginning of homework, takes an extra long time to complete homework or rushes through homework, doesn't always finish homework.
- Difficulty with maintaining attention: has trouble focusing on task and staying with task, daydreams, loses attention quickly, is easily distracted, "fiddles" with everything on the desk.

We are describing those individuals who, after their position has been criticized or corrected, slip right back into the position or move into another socially unacceptable one. The sitting positions that are socially acceptable are very uncomfortable to the person fighting the pull of the STNR.

When we were teachers working with children in the classroom, we would tap them on their shoulders time after time and politely say, "Sit up straight. Slouching is bad for your spine." They would reply that they were more comfortable in that slouching position. Very presumptuously, we would respond, "No, you're not. I'm the teacher, and I know how you are comfortable. Now, sit up straight." How sad that we were unable to believe the children's words or understand their body language. Of course, we didn't know about the STNR then.

If your child is having problems with sitting and/or paying attention consider the possibility that the major problem may be an immature STNR. Become a detective: look for clues; analyze the child's body positions.

Read on to discover the psychological consequences of the immature STNR.

4. Psychological Consequences of an Immature STNR

Our clinical experience has convinced us that most STNR children do *not* have primary psychological problems. However, many of them do suffer psychological consequences caused by the interference of the STNR and by the misdiagnosis and mistreatment of the real problem—the STNR. An immature STNR can cause psychological interference with academic performance and social interaction. Although basic intelligence is not affected by an immature STNR, interference by the STNR in school and social situations can create psychological consequences.

If the STNR stays at an immature level, it can greatly interfere with specific and general coordination tasks, frequently generating the following emotional and psychological consequences:

- poor peer relationships
- low self-esteem
- frustration, avoidance, and aggression
- inflexibility

Poor Peer Relationships

An immature STNR can wreak havoc with children's social lives. It can interfere with children's social interactions on the playground, in the classroom, and after school. Because their motor skills are in-adequate, STNR children frequently are not invited to play with other children, do not have the desire to play with them, or do not have time to play. These children may appear lazy and unmotivated, but we do not believe that STNR children are avoiding play because they are lazy or uninterested. In school, many STNR children do not join their peers in play and other social interaction at recess time be-cause they have to stay in the classroom to finish the work that they were unable to finish in the time that their peers found sufficient. Af-ter school, they don't get to play with their neighborhood friends, ei-ther, because they are usually made to start on their homework as soon as they get home, since their parents know from experience that homework tasks take them a considerable length of time to com-plete. Many are at their desks or at the kitchen table morning, noon, and into the night because they must put so much effort into accom-plishing even unsatisfactory schoolwork.

Many others avoid play that involves activities that are extremely difficult for them. When children express intense dislike for a partic-ular task or activity, or lack of interest in it, they usually are not good at it, or they have to put forth so much effort that it's not worth the trouble to them. They quickly learn to avoid activities at which they can't succeed with a reasonable amount of effort. A case in point concerns a young boy named Mark.

When we first met him, Mark was five years old, extremely bright, and one of the most gifted readers we have ever known. (His read-ing and comprehension were at least at the twelfth grade level!) We handed him a senior literature book and opened it at random. Mark proceeded to read fluently, and he also understood what he read; however, he didn't like to run, and he couldn't ride a bike. Mark told us he didn't like his Big Wheel. (His parents told us he did not know how to ride it.) He told us he did not like to play ball with the neighborhood children, and when we tried to play pitch and catch with him, we knew why. He rarely went out of the house, and even more rarely interacted with the neighborhood children, stating that he preferred to stay in and read. Wouldn't it seem great to have a five-year-old who devoted most of his time to reading? No, not when it's at the expense of other important development. Justifiably pleased with Mark's reading ability, his parents were, nevertheless, seriously concerned about his lack of social and motoric development. While they were not trying to force Mark to be an athlete, they knew the importance of physical activity for health, social development, and just plain childhood fun.

Mark's mother, a pediatrician, was very open to a variety of explanations of behavior. She could accept explanations other than blaming the child, and she could accept forms of treatment other than prescribing drugs. (Her openness was possibly due to the fact that she was trained in England.)

After appropriate testing, we determined that although Mark was very bright intellectually, he was on the other end of the scale motorically. He was actually what some people would call "motorically retarded." When he ran, which was seldom, he looked like the scarecrow in *The Wizard of Oz*—arms and legs going in all directions.

Mark had done very little crawling as a baby, and he had walked early. His parents knew that crawling was an important part of normal development. They were unaware, however, of the potential problems caused by missing or shortening the crawling stage. We assigned exercises designed to mature the STNR. Mark and his parents worked diligently at this program.

Then one day his mother called to tell us that Mark had just had the second happiest day of his life (the first was when he had learned to read). She said that the previous day, when he had come shrieking in the back door, she was afraid he had broken an arm or cracked his head. It took her a few minutes to calm him down to find the reason for his excitement. He wasn't hurt; he was happy. He had just ridden his Big Wheel for the first time! He dashed back out to ". . . ride bikes . . ." with the children next door. His parents were barely able to get him back inside for dinner.

Mark had successfully completed the STNR exercise program, and his STNR had matured. Now, Mark was easily able to enjoy the fun of childhood and to continue his love affair with reading.

If some STNR children exclude themselves from specific games and play activities, other STNR children are excluded by their peers. Some STNR children would like to participate, even though their skills are deficient, but they are seldom invited, and they are often not even allowed into group activities. Frequently, these STNR children are rejected because their skills are so poor that no one wants them on the team.

Some STNR children are rejected because they have such poor control of their bodies. Their muscle action is very inconsistent, and they "read" it very poorly. What they intend to be enthusiastic pats-on-the-back may become clumsy shoves. When these children mean to give only a playful push, the other youngster frequently ends up on the ground. The shover may be as surprised as the "shovee," but the STNR child's protest that "I didn't mean to push him that hard!" is not easy to believe unless one realizes that because of the immature STNR these children truly have extremely poor motor control and little awareness of their muscle force.

STNR children may also give the impression that they are not interested in a game because of the difficulties they experience in sitting in the upright posture that most people interpret as indicating alertness and interest. Instead, they may slouch or "wallow" on the ground, on the bench, or in the dugout because sitting still is so difficult for them. They look "clumsy," "lazy," and "unmotivated," so they are chosen last by players and coaches alike. Children should not have to live with such labels. Instead of using "clumsy," "lazy," and "unmotivated" as labels, we see these behaviors as clues. When these children comment, "I don't like baseball," or another sport from which they have been excluded, it is often an attempt to cover up the exclusion, whether it has come from peers, adults, or the STNR child as a self-protective measure. An immature STNR can wreak havoc with a child's social life.

Poor peer relationships can be a psychological consequence of an immature STNR.

Low Self-Esteem

STNR children rarely achieve success easily, and frequently don't achieve success at all. Limited success tends to produce low self-esteem. Dr. Miriam Bender (1997) estimates that STNR children have to use at least *ten times* the amount of energy and effort as do children without the immature STNR. Even when they continue to work "ten times harder," the quality and quantity of their work are often inferior, if acceptable at all. STNR children rarely compete well academically or athletically. Inevitably, the unfavorable comparison to their friends is demoralizing. Comments such as the following are all too frequent in the lives of STNR children:

"You've got to try harder!"
"You're just stupid!"
"Why are you so lazy?"
"Why can't you keep up with Jimmy?"

Comments such as these are devastating to self-esteem. We are reminded of the story of a professor of psychology.

The professor entered his classroom one day with a large piece of paper pinned to his shirt. On the paper were the letters IALAC. The professor announced that the piece of paper represented his self-esteem. The letters meant "I am loved and caring."

"Now," he said, "as the day goes on, if I hear a negative comment, it takes a little bit out of me. Pretend I am a young child. As I come downstairs for breakfast, my mother says, 'I looked at your homework. It's very sloppy. You'll have to do it over before you turn it in.'" And the professor reached up and tore off a piece of the IALAC paper pinned to his shirt.

"Then," he continued, "at school the teacher looks at me and says, 'Please sit up straight—you look so lazy!'" And the professor reached up and tore off another piece of the paper pinned to his shirt.

"Now," he said, "imagine if these comments continue all day . . .

"We don't want him on our team.'
"There isn't anyone left to choose from, so I guess we'll take you.'
"Look at this spelling paper—what a mess!'"

Each time a negative comment was made, the professor tore another piece from his IALAC paper, which became smaller and smaller and smaller.

"Now," said the professor, "by the time I get home and ready for bed"—and he took the pin from his shirt and held it up, and his students all stared at the bare pin—"*this* is all that's left." He made the point the self-esteem, whether it's high or low, is formed every day, every minute, with every comment.

Eventually, STNR children begin to believe that these negative comments are accurate. They will even begin to make negative comments about themselves before other people can. They often develop a defeatist attitude, figuring, "Why should I even bother trying?" In many cases these children even begin to question their own intelligence. They doubt that they can be as smart as other children if they have to work so hard on everyday tasks.

Stephen, a fifth-grade boy, had an assignment of fifty math problems. Working diligently, he copied twenty-five of them. Realizing that his time was running out, he worked the twenty-five problems, and he got twenty-four correct out of the twenty-five. Generally, twenty-four out of twenty-five would be at least an A-. What grade do you think *he* got? You're right! He got an F! The teacher reasoned that Stephen had correctly worked only twenty-four of fifty. The fact that he was correct in 96 percent of what he completed was ignored. It does not take bright children very long to figure, "If I'm going to get an F no matter how hard I work, why bother knocking myself out? I must really be stupid!"

*Low self-esteem can be a psychological consequence of an imma-
ture STNR.*

Frustration, Avoidance,
and Aggression

In many typical, everyday situations, parents of STNR children
are frequently labeled "too permissive" and the children themselves
as "willfully misbehaving." Everyday society surrounds children with
situations that require them to sit down, sit up straight, sit still, pay
attention, write neatly and quickly, play ball, eat in a mannerly fashion, ride a bicycle, play a musical instrument, and color *inside* the
lines. Most children meet these requirements with relative ease, with
general success, usually with pleasure, and frequently with joy. STNR
children meet these requirements, if they are able to meet them at all,
only through extreme effort, with minimal success, usually with little pleasure, and rarely with anything approaching joy. It is easy to
see how everybody involved can become frustrated and irritable.
Frustration seems inevitable for STNR children and for all who have
to deal with them.

There are two basic causes for this frustration:

- STNR children cannot easily meet society's demands for maintaining attention, coordinated sitting, standing, writing, eating,
  and playing.
- Most parents, teachers, and other professionals do not know
  about the immature STNR and, therefore, continue to demand
  abilities and coordination that are unavailable to STNR children.

For example, children with an immature STNR frequently have
difficulty learning to ride a bicycle. In our society, there is extreme
peer pressure to ride a bike in order to be one of the crowd. Some
STNR children will eventually give up trying to learn after repeated

failures and many tears. Others will persist through the numerous cuts and bruises and eventually will be able to join their friends on bikes. It is probably worth the effort, but it is certainly not easy for them. (Some STNR children have learned that turning their handlebars or front wheels around makes it easier to keep their arms straight while they are bending their knees to pedal. They don't know why it's easier; they just know that it is.)

Parents agonize along with their children, watching their valiant but often futile efforts to succeed in tasks that most children master fairly easily. However, if the agony of defeat is shared, so—when it comes—is the ecstasy of success. One client's mother called us after working with her daughter on our STNR exercise program. She told us that her husband was standing in the yard crying; she was close to tears herself. After years of being unable to ride a bicycle, their ten-year-old daughter was finally wobbling down the driveway on her bicycle for the first time. We shared their tears of joy. A small matter, riding a bike? . . . Not in the everyday life of a ten-year-old.

Children learn early to avoid tasks at which they cannot succeed as quickly and easily as other children. No one enjoys being made fun of. Consequently, children with an immature STNR will either have to work ten times harder to achieve at an acceptable level, or they will "choose" not to participate, usually giving excuses like the following ones:

"I don't like baseball (football, basketball, etc.) anyway."

"I'd rather keep score than play."

"I'm too tired to play."

"Baseball (football, basketball, etc.) is dumb . . . a waste of time . . . borrrrring."

"I'd rather watch TV . . . read . . . play with my cars . . . build models. . . ."

We have learned to question these "logical" excuses. Are they legitimate reasons or are they avoidance tactics? We are not saying that everyone has to practice in a sport in order to be a happy, healthy, well-rounded individual. Nor are we saying that a child should not read or watch TV or build models. We are saying that a variety of types of activities—individual and group, nonphysical and physical—is important. Individual activities contribute to personal development; group activities are essential for socialization. Children who entertain themselves *primarily* in nonphysical, solitary activities generally do so because they are unsuccessful in physically interactive group games.

The frustration of STNR children will often lead to avoidance and withdrawal tactics—or to confrontation and aggression. These children cannot understand, any more than some adults can, why many simple tasks seem so difficult for them. Some STNR children withdraw from or resist participation in activities that they have previously failed or that they find newly threatening. They may claim that they do not participate in these activities because they "hate" them. Other children continue to struggle, working harder than their peers, and often express their frustration through anger, excuses, or demonstrations of poor sportsmanship.

Frustration, avoidance, and aggression can be psychological consequences of an immature STNR.

Inflexibility

Often, STNR children attempt to increase their chances for success by imposing very rigid rules on themselves and their surroundings. From fear of failing totally, they may become extremely inflexible, not daring to vary one smidgen from a routine that they have found at least somewhat successful.

A teacher called us one day and asked that we come observe her little Jamie, a third grader, who was puzzling her. Ordinarily Jamie was very cooperative, she told us, but sometimes he just refused to do certain tasks, and she couldn't find the reason for his apparent obstinacy. (We commended her for not jumping to the conclusion that Jamie was just being obnoxious, but that there had to be a reason for his behavior.)

We went over to the classroom and observed for a few days, immediately noticing Jamie's STNR sitting postures. He worked slowly, but was cooperative—unless some aspect of the day was changed or out of its usual order. If the reading class was supposed to come before the arithmetic class, he seemed confused and upset if the teacher reversed the order and wanted to do arithmetic first.

We suggested to the teacher that, because of the STNR, Jamie was exerting all his energy just sitting at his desk, trying to be comfortable in any position that the teacher would allow. STNR children can sometimes manage to function in the security of a structured, predictable environment, but they have no energy left over for any change in the routine. Anything out of the ordinary can cause STNR children to balk and refuse to change.

When we talked with his mother, she told us that he was the same at home. His belongings had to be arranged in a particular way, and any deviation would "send him into orbit." Often STNR children tend to be very messy and disorganized, but when they have acquired some confidence and sense of security in structure, they are really structured to the point of being inflexible.

When STNR children have gained some degree of success in sports, they frequently resist changing their stances, their grips, or the way they release the ball, even if the coach assures them that the new form will contribute to better performance. To the amazement of others, they may choose to stick with a familiar approach that has been totally unsuccessful, rather than to try something new.

Unfortunately, the inflexibility they adopt to *lessen* their frustration often serves to *compound* their frustration. They lock themselves in to using inadequate but familiar methods for solving daily problems, and lock themselves out of trying new methods that are potentially better.

We were asked to visit a second-grade classroom to observe Larry. Because his printing was slow, laborious, and somewhat messy, the teacher had thought that Larry would welcome moving on to cursive writing. This was not the case. Ever since she had introduced cursive writing to the class, Larry had been having tantrums during writing time. He even got sick to his stomach and threw up during one writing session.

It didn't take long for us to recognize some of Larry's classic STNR characteristics: feet wrapped around the chair legs, writing for short periods of time. We even noticed the "writer's bump" on his finger . . . and he was only in the second grade!

Some children can't verbalize what they are thinking or feeling, but Larry was somewhat able to do so. When we asked Larry why he didn't like the new cursive writing, he said, "I'm *just* getting the hang of printing!" With great effort, he had learned to print, although not neatly or quickly. At this point, he was extremely unwilling to take on the new task of cursive writing when printing got the job done.

Because of their fear of trying something new, STNR children are often labeled as uncompromising and uncooperative, and always wanting to have their own way.

Inflexibility can be a psychological consequence of an immature STNR.

If your child is having problems with poor peer relationships, low self-esteem, frustration, avoidance, aggression, or inflexibility, consider that the major problem may be an immature STNR, rather than a primary psychological problem.

Read on to discover how the immature STNR can cause problems in school, in sports, at home, and in public settings.

PART TWO

How to Work Around the Real Problem

If, through your detective work, you have determined that someone you know (yourself, your child, or your spouse, for example) has an immature STNR, there are two ways of dealing with the problem: circumventions and interventions.

Circumventions: methods for working *around* a problem.

Interventions: methods for working *through* a problem, actually solving it.

In general, interventions are obviously more desirable than circumventions. We truly thank God that, because of Dr. Miriam Bender's work (see the discussions in the preface and introduction), interventions are available for maturing the STNR. However, interventions require several months to implement. Consequently, we will first discuss circumventions, which you can begin even as you read this chapter, and which you can continue as you provide interventions for an immature STNR.

We are recommending acceptance of the circumventions that are described in chapters 5 through 8, depending on what the people involved can tolerate. We are recommending flexibility, not chaos. Children with an immature STNR are not the only ones with rights—other people have rights, too. For example, we might suggest accepting a child's preference for standing or lying down in certain situations. However, we would not expect everyone to accept the child's standing on the couch to watch TV or lying in the aisle at the movies.

Often, STNR children do not realize that they are circumventing—working around a problem. They do not even realize that they *have* a problem. Because people have only themselves as reference points, they do not really know how difficult—or easy—a task is for other people. STNR children just know that their lives require a great deal of effort. While effort is highly regarded and rewarded in our society, the effort involved in circumvention is a strain and often a drain of energy. Nevertheless, in an effort to cope, most STNR children will automatically devise or come up with some kind of circumvention.

STNR children frequently employ one or both of the following circumventions at home, in school, and in the community (e.g., movies, places of worship, sporting events):

- They will seek postural comfort by sitting in a variety of positions, standing, or lying down.
- They will avoid situations that are difficult or unpleasant for them.

STNR children give ample evidence that they *need* these circumventions by their persistence in using them. *We strongly recommend that you accept the basic need for these circumventions.* But that's not enough! In order to be most productive, STNR children need your help and support in implementing their coping mechanisms.

If you have not already read Part One of this book, be sure to go back and read it before looking at the following chapters. The material that follows will be much more meaningful to you if you have read the preceding four chapters. The following chapters describe the kinds of problems STNR children have and offer circumventions for them at school, in sports, at home, and in the community. These circumventions will help STNR children benefit as much as possible from their efforts and will make their lives easier and happier. Remember that these circumventions are suggestions for *working around* the interfering effects of an immature STNR. These circumventions can be and should be implemented immediately for the STNR child at school, at home, and away from home. These circumventions can bring great relief from frustration, physical tension, fatigue, and discomfort, and they can greatly enhance attention span, efficiency, ease in writing, cooperation, and self-esteem.

5. School Problems

How does the immature STNR interfere with schoolwork? We find that many children are not doing well in school simply because they don't do their writing assignments well (or at all). It has been our experience that many children having difficulties in school do not have basic difficulties understanding the material. Their basic problems are with sitting still, maintaining attention, and writing—all hampered by the immature STNR. "Some educational weaknesses can be traced directly to inadequate reflex development. For example, Jane Field (1989, 1990) explains how postural difficulties in handwriting are traced to uninhibited asymmetric and symmetric tonic neck reflexes." (Anderson 1999, p. 77)

The educational implications of abnormal activity of the STNR can be quite complex and far-reaching. Not all academic problems result from an immature STNR, of course, but many academic problems are compounded by this reflex's interference. Its presence in the immature state controls the pattern of muscular tension in the child's arms and legs in relation to head movements. Movement of any one of the three involved body parts elicits the reflex response in the other two parts. These involuntary movements interfere with the child's gaining control over the body; that is, the body still controls the child.

All movements that the child makes must be performed within the constricting influence of the STNR. The child must almost consciously attend to even simple motor acts. The immature reflex generally hampers the production of rhythmic, coordinated movement as well as the ability to pay attention easily, and specifically interferes with the postures generally required for reading and writing.

An immature STNR makes it very difficult for the child to sit at a desk in the "correct sitting position," with elbows and hips bent at the same time. Under the influence of the reflex, the neck and elbows want to straighten in opposition to the bending of the legs, and vice versa. Consequently, when the child bends his or her arms to write or to hold a book for reading, the legs tend to straighten. Frequently STNR children sit in a slouched position with their legs stretched out in front of them. Many teachers consider this position "bad for the spine," "lazy," and a hindrance to the child's work. These teachers do not realize that this position is actually comfortable for the child with an immature STNR because the arms and neck are not "fighting" with the position of the hips and legs.

When STNR children are not allowed to sit in the slouched position, they frequently become "foot sitters," sitting in their chairs with their feet and legs tucked under their own bodies. This position "locks" the feet so that the arms and neck can bend while the legs are also bent. Another favorite posture for such children is sitting with their feet hooked around the legs of the chair. While these positions do not make the child truly comfortable, they do enable the STNR child to stay seated for a while.

Many children with an immature STNR are called ADHD. They have extreme difficulty sitting still for long periods of time in the "proper sitting position" and in maintaining attention. They may stand up and sit down repeatedly in order to relieve the tension caused by the reflex. STNR children, also, usually have poor penmanship. Their written work is laboriously produced, with poor letter formation, and they hold the writing implement in a rigid or awkward manner. Every shift of the arm while writing also causes a change in the tension of the neck and hips; consequently, these children write in a constricted, restricted, and cramped position to avoid muscular changes. Copying from the board to a paper on the desk is an especially difficult task because the child has to contend with the reflex effects of frequent positional changes in the neck and arm. Children who combat these problems may write laboriously, almost drawing their letters. Although their finished products may look good, the time and effort expended are disproportionately high. If the production of the paper takes significantly longer than it does for other children, the action is inefficient even if the paper looks well done. As discussed in chapter 2, Dr. Bender's research indicates that at least 75 percent of children with academic or behavioral problems have an immature STNR as a contributing factor. This means that the basic problem for many children who are failing academically may come from the difficulties they experience with the *mechanics* of learning, such as handwriting and copying material from a chalkboard, rather than from the mental effort required.

In spelling, for example, the STNR child's poor performance may more often be caused by the physical effort required of the child and the discomfort it produces than by the child's lack of spelling skill. Many of these children can pass a spelling test if they are allowed to do it orally rather than having to write the words.

In arithmetic, children with an immature STNR frequently experience more difficulty in copying the problems from a book or from the board than in comprehending the concepts and performing the computations. Often they expend more energy in trying to accomplish the physical act of copying problems and writing answers than they do in calculation. Frequently, these children will complete the first part of an assignment. However, as their discomfort increases and they exhaust themselves by shifting and reshifting their positions in an effort to make themselves comfortable and get the work done, they will not finish the assignment. Maintaining consistent attention throughout this ordeal is really impossible. Sometimes, they will complete the assignment by putting just any answer on the paper in order to hand in a "finished" product. As STNR children grow older and accumulate more and more experiences of failure, they tend to avoid written work as much as possible, with the result that they often appear lazy and totally uninterested in their schoolwork.

After more than thirty years of clinical experience involving the reading of countless school records; talking to parents, teachers, school psychologists, and doctors; and interpreting test results, we are convinced that the academic and behavioral problems of children are rarely diagnosed properly. Many of these children are called lazy or slow; some are called "all boy," whatever that means; they are told that they are not trying hard enough. We think that these traditional interpretations are grossly inaccurate. The interfering effects of the immature STNR provide a more complete and satisfactory explanation for the behavior and performance of these children. The immature STNR causes or adds to the problems of most children who are struggling in school. Additionally, some STNR children may perform well in school, but only at the expense of a tremendous amount of time, effort, and energy: *they work too hard for the grades they get.*

The immature reflex can seriously interfere in many academic areas. Understanding the STNR interference provides a totally new

The Importance of Early Motor Development

Based on her study of sensory and motor integration, Jean Ayres hypothesized (Ayres 1972) that ability in reading must be quite dependent on mechanisms in the brain that help maintain normal posture. She derived this hypothesis from the fact that children who experience certain kinds of difficulties in integrating the functions of the two hemispheres of the brain also have difficulty integrating the motor functions of the two sides of the body. Ayres found that "this problem is ameliorated when postural mechanisms are normalized."

The Emory University study of the role of body reflexes and motor skills in learning disabilities (Freides et al. 1980) concluded that appropriate remediation "would first inhibit the interfering symmetric tonic neck reflex, and these procedures might include activities remote from usual classroom techniques."

and different explanation for some traditionally unacceptable behaviors and misunderstood difficulties. It has been our experience that it is easier to provide help for STNR children when parents and teachers really understand how this reflex interferes with children's efforts and success.

In dealing with these children, the most important thing to remember is that they are not willfully being overactive, not purposely avoiding their assignments, not intentionally trying your patience. What they are asked to do may be ten times more difficult for STNR children than for children without these reflex interferences. Under the conditions usually imposed upon them, they cannot manage certain tasks without a tremendous amount of effort. It is necessary for teachers to try to help STNR children circumvent their problems. *These children should not be penalized for something not under their control*.

We do not ask that responsibilities be lessened for STNR children, since that is not in their best interest. We do request that these children be allowed to express ideas in alternative methods that come as easily to them as writing does to children who do not have to cope with the interference of an immature STNR. Then the work that they produce is more likely to be indicative of what the children really know, without being hidden or stifled by the additional chore of writing.

Knowledge of the immature STNR provides explanations, not excuses, for easily misunderstood behavior.

Comfort and Attention Span

How do you think continuous movement or the need to move affects the STNR child's attention span? Paying attention is very difficult while constantly moving in an effort to get comfortable or while managing to sit still but in an uncomfortable position. Some children have to use most of their effort and energy trying to sit still; they have very little energy left for listening to the teacher or doing their work.

Think back to the position we asked you to assume at the beginning of this book, in the spelling test. How good would your reading comprehension be at this point if you were still maintaining that position? Not so hot? You would be expending most of your energy maintaining your position, rather than directing your attention toward this interesting material.

Some STNR children can't sit still even when they try, so they move around, trying to get comfortable. Many of these children make so much noise, or distract themselves so much with moving around, that they interfere with their own listening.

> One little girl, Beth, did very poorly on a listening test we gave her. Even though she was seated during the testing, her feet were in constant motion. We suspected that Beth's antsiness and the noise she herself was making contributed to her low score on the test. We allowed Beth to stand, which she did quietly, and gave her another form of the test. Under these conditions, Beth scored much better on the listening test. Her basic listening problem was self-distracting noise and motion, rather than a hearing loss. She was doing poorly in listening because she was doing so poorly in sitting quietly.

Children can create so much noise and distraction moving around trying to get comfortable that they really do not hear the teacher. This is just one example of many possible interfering effects of the immature STNR.

Comfort and Attention-Span Circumventions

The following circumventions will allow STNR children to pay closer attention for a longer period of time by making them more comfortable.

- *Allow postural freedom.* Sitting in a variety of positions, standing, lying down, getting up and down occasionally, running errands, walking around occasionally (this does not include looking over other children's shoulders or elbowing friends).
- Modify the situation to help the STNR child get comfortable (as in the following examples):

- Provide "rolling desks." One innovative teacher helped an antsy seventh-grader by obtaining a tall cart on wheels from a beauty salon. The student stood at this unique "desk" in the back of the room, moving at will. He became much more productive. The other students quickly adjusted to this arrangement, finding it much less disruptive than his previous antsiness.
  - Trade a "walker" for a "talker." If it really bothers you to have a student walk around the classroom, trade with another teacher who is bothered more by a talker. Such trades can provide relief for all concerned.
- Be creative and open to new ideas.
- *Reject* the shortsighted, limiting, uninformed, thoughtless, misguided, weak excuse, "If we do it for one, we have to do it for everybody." (Does everyone in the class have to wear glasses if only one or two need them?)
- Allow recess time. If recess is not scheduled, *provide it. Do not keep students in from recess to finish writing assignments.*
- Be as pleasant and patient as possible.

Writing (Dysgraphia)

Writing is usually extremely difficult for STNR children. The writing done by STNR children usually looks one of two ways:

- Most often, it is very messy, having been written in a hurry to get it over with, or just to keep up with the rest of the class. Sometimes it is messy-looking even when the child has spent a great deal of time on it.
- Occasionally it appears very neat and may even be displayed on the bulletin board. However, this neatness is usually achieved at great expense of time, effort, and energy.

When a child comes to our clinic, one of the first things we ask about is penmanship. Messy writing very often indicates the involvement of an immature STNR. However, if the writing is neat, we are pleased for the child, but have learned to ask a second question, "How long did it take?" One teacher replied, "Oh, he missed two recesses and stayed in at lunch, but after all, he's such a perfectionist." Here was a good teacher giving her student extra time, but totally misinterpreting why he needed it. She didn't know about the immature STNR and its effects on handwriting.

Parents and teachers should communicate more frequently about the amount of time children spend on homework. Often, teachers have no idea of the amount of time that it takes STNR children to do their homework. Teachers have only the finished product to judge, and have no knowledge of the process involved, particularly the amount of time, effort, and energy that an STNR child expends to produce even minimally acceptable work.

On one occasion, we went to a school counseling meeting for Jimmy, a fourth grader. When the teacher arrived, Jimmy's mother "lit into" her, almost shouting. "How can you give a child four hours of homework every night? He doesn't have any time for anything but schoolwork!" The teacher was amazed, and when she had the opportunity to speak, she said that most of the homework should not take more than forty-five minutes to an hour *in total*. As it turned out, Jimmy's writing was laborious; he was constantly getting up and sitting down in an effort to get comfortable and complete his work, and his assignments took much longer than the teacher would have expected. Using the reflex test, we tested Jimmy and found that the STNR was significantly bothering him. We gave the teacher some suggestions for circumventions and worked with the parents to mature the reflex.

We understand that, at home, parents may not realize what should be a reasonable amount of time for children to be spending on their homework. The average parent often does not have an accurate frame of reference for the amount of time a given assignment should take. Nor do STNR children have an accurate frame of reference; they only know how long and hard they have to work when the other kids are playing or watching TV. The time involved in doing an assignment can be a good clue to the presence of an immature STNR.

However, while time can easily be measured, *it is impossible to determine the amount of effort* that goes into an assignment. The amount of time spent may not reflect the amount of effort put forth. Some STNR children may put forth great effort but may not be able to sustain it for an extended amount of time. They often look as if they don't care or aren't trying because they don't work for very long. These children usually get very little sympathy and even less help.

On the other hand, the effort some children expend is more obvious. Parents and teachers are more likely to agonize and sympathize with the STNR children who perspire, grimace, and spend hours on writing assignments, and who cry from frustration. The irony of all of this is that our society usually regards as admirable the spending of excessive amounts of time and effort on schoolwork. One mother proudly told us, "My son is such a perfectionist. He did his assignment twenty times until it was without a mistake!" How sad we think that is! A child with at least average intelligence shouldn't have to do an assignment twenty times to get it right.

These STNR children can't seem to win no matter what they do. If they don't complete their assignments, they get F's; if they do complete them, it takes forever. We have found that some children have figured out that their self-esteem is greater if they don't even *do* an assignment: If they get an F, they seem to think it is better to say, "I didn't even try," than to say that they worked like crazy and still got an F. It must seem to them that their entire childhood is spent on school tasks—morning, noon, and night. They have little time simply to be children and play.

We are certainly not saying that children should not be expected to spend some time and effort on schoolwork, but we strongly object to their having to spend so much time and effort on tasks that should be done more easily and automatically. The average child should be able to complete an average amount of work in an average length of time. Parents and teachers need to be alert to the quantity of time involved as well as the quality of work.

Writing is a very difficult chore for STNR children. The immature STNR interferes with, but does not prevent, writing. (It is inhibitive, not prohibitive.) Children with this reflex immaturity can sit up straight, but *not comfortably;* they can write, but *not easily.* Remember that the immature STNR essentially keeps the neck, arms, and legs "tied" together. Movement of any one of these parts causes muscular reaction in the other two parts; STNR children are under constant physical stress. It is as if thick rubber bands are pulling their arms straight out when these children are sitting "properly." They can pull their arms in to write, but only with great effort. Many of these STNR children are fatigued by ten o'clock in the morning because of the extra effort and energy they expend in writing tasks.

Dr. Miriam Bender (1997) estimates that STNR children use at least *ten times* as much energy as do children without these problems, and yet these are the children frequently referred to as lazy or lacking in motivation because they don't finish their work. Consider the child who has three worksheets to complete for a morning's work. If this child has an immature STNR, a three-page assignment represents the same amount of work as *thirty* pages for a child whose efforts are not impeded by an immature STNR—an overwhelming task. Is it any wonder that these children have desks filled with half-completed work? Some STNR children are so physically tired from copying math problems or English exercises from the board or from books to their papers that they have no energy left for doing the assignment. Others take so long in the copying that there is no time left to work the problems. By the time they are in junior high or high school, many STNR children have learned that it is pointless even to begin a writing assignment. One of our bright young clients described his problem very well: "I can do the brain work; I just can't copy."

One time, we did a presentation for a group of teachers at an elementary school. We explained how the immature reflex causes STNR children to work ten times harder than most children, sometimes still not producing work reflective of their intelligence. The principal of the school followed us out to our car. It was obvious that he did not mean to compliment us when he said, "You just want to make life easy for these kids." We said, "That's right!" Life and school can be frustrating and difficult enough for children. Why make it harder?

Another youngster we were testing was a third grader named Joey. When asked to take a spelling test, he politely announced, "I don't do spelling." None of our professional charms could coax him into taking the spelling test. He had never passed a written spelling test and firmly refused to enter into what he considered a no-win situation. He finally said, "Just give me an F, and let's get on with it."

Because of the immature STNR, writing was really difficult for him. Joey was one of those children who know how to spell all the words orally on Thursday night but fail the written test on Friday morning. Although Joey appeared to have a spelling problem, it was really the writing he couldn't do, not the spelling. We admired his determination to protect his self-esteem. While a grade of F certainly did not *raise* his self-esteem, getting an F for no output of energy was not so demoralizing as getting an F after working really hard.

In spite of the immature STNR, some children try to keep up with their writing. Many of them experience such muscular tension while gripping their pencils that they frequently have to put their pencils down and shake their hands to stimulate circulation in their fingers. Some will stop writing and rest awhile; they are often accused of daydreaming, wasting time, and being inattentive when, in fact, their real problem is writer's cramp.

Another clue to the presence of the immature STNR is the "death grip" some of these children get on their pencils in an attempt to bring their writing under their control. Many of these STNR children develop a "writer's bump" on their fingers from the incredible pressure they put on their pencils. Still others, in an effort to avoid the pressure of the "death grip," hold the pencil in every fashion other than the "correct" way.

Greg, a fourth-grade child, told us that he wrote with his right hand until it got too tired. Then he switched his pencil to his left hand and continued his writing, although he was the only one who could read it. When his right hand was sufficiently rested, he put the pencil back in it, erased what he had done with his left hand,

and rewrote it with his right. We asked Greg why he bothered to write with his left hand instead of just resting for a while. He said he had tried that, but his teacher had told him to quit goofing off and to keep working.

Greg had been referred to us because a truly conscientious teacher felt that he was not working hard enough. Here he was, writing with both hands, and the teacher still kept telling him, "Try a little harder." How much harder can you try than to write with both hands?

This type of effort from a child often goes unrecognized or ignored because the finished product looks so bad. The child is scolded for messy work and told to do it over because he "obviously did not spend much time or effort on that."

You can see that the "tricky" aspect of this reflex is that when STNR children are fresh and rested, in the morning, they can fight the pull of the STNR and keep up with the work for a while. It is confusing to the teacher and children when, two hours later, the quality of the work greatly diminishes as the children become more and more fatigued from having to cope with the reflex. Who can blame a teacher for considering it a duty to encourage a child to maintain the higher quality of work? However, the STNR child's daily supply of energy is frequently "used up" by noon.

One boy we were testing used up his energy supply for writing in the first five minutes. Rick, who was going into junior high school, wrote ten words in a spelling quiz for us, and then rested for a few minutes. His writing was legible, but certainly would not have received a penmanship award. [See figure 5.1.] After a short break, we had him begin another list of ten words. He wrote three words, and his writing deteriorated into a total mess. This boy could write thirteen words, and then he "had had it." His comment was, "Please. No more writing." Can you imagine how difficult junior high school and college might be for such a boy? (By the way, Rick's I.Q. was 135—in the superior range.)

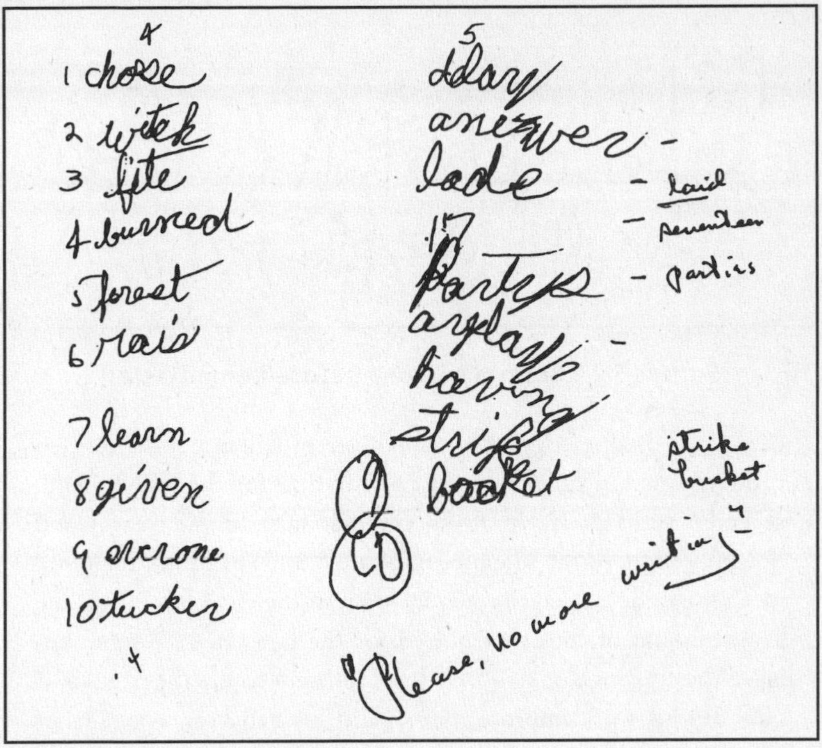

FIGURE 5.1. **Rick's Paper**

Another example of the confusion caused by the interference of the STNR on written work is illustrated by the story of Ronnie, a first-grade boy referred to us.

Ronnie's teacher stated that she did not think he was mentally handicapped, but that his written work was of such low quality that she could not be sure. Ronnie had finished an entire year of kindergarten and a full semester of first grade. A battery of tests—I.Q., reflex, reading, math—revealed that his only major problem was the immature STNR. His I.Q. was 115, classifying him as above average in intelligence.

For one of the tests, Ronnie was asked to copy the alphabet from the chalkboard to his paper. This task took him fifteen min

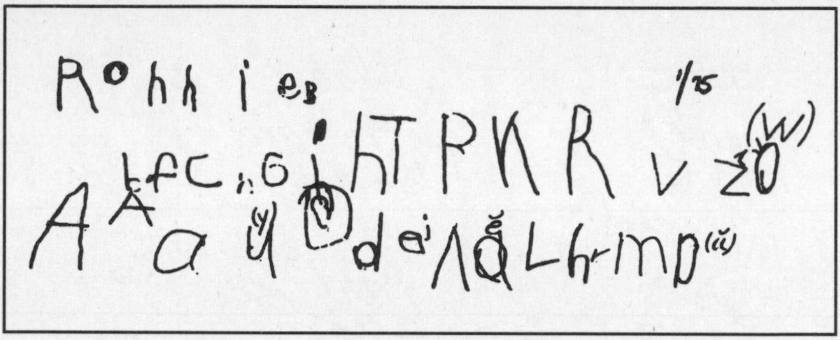

FIGURE 5.2. Ronnie's Paper Before Remediation

utes of labored writing. As you can see in figure 5.2, his written product was pitiful. We began remediation for the STNR, and, several months later, with no special help in writing, he easily and quickly produced the sentence in figure 5.3. (We did not turn him into a poet; he copied the sentences from the chalkboard.) In the same amount of time as required for the first effort, Ronnie finished the copying and had time left over to decorate the page. Not only did his work improve, but so did his behavior. His teacher called us and said she was trying to figure out what was so different about the last few weeks of school. She finally realized that she was no longer telling Ronnie to sit down and do his work thirty or forty times a day. Now when she called his name, it was with a compli-

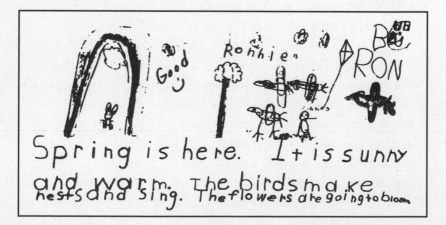

FIGURE 5.3. Ronnie's Paper After Remediation

ment. Ronnie was as delighted as the teacher was. The maturation of the STNR had improved his behavior as well as his writing.

For children still fighting the immature STNR, writing continues to be a problem. Some resist even beginning their papers—putting it off, and putting it off, and putting it off, to the frustration of their parents and teachers. When they are asked why they put off starting their assignments, most children say they don't know. But *we* know. Because of the immature STNR, their writing is laborious and inefficient. They can maintain the effort required to work ten times as hard as anyone else for only so long. If these STNR children finally do begin, many will stop before completing the assignment, and others will have run out of time. A few will struggle on to the finish, almost too tired to feel pleasure in their accomplishment.

Writing is really difficult for STNR children.

Writing Circumventions

The following circumventions will enable STNR children to more easily express themselves in writing. (Remember: these are circumventions for the STNR, not techniques for teaching writing.)

- Allow *postural freedom*.
- Require less writing.
    - Give shorter writing assignments.
    - Allow children to underline or circle answers rather than writing them out.
    - Allow children to give oral responses to the teacher or an aide, or into a tape recorder.
    - Accept single-word answers rather than complete sentences.
    - Allow children to substitute oral book reports and/or projects for written assignments.
    - Allow chalkboard work as an alternative to paperwork.
    - Accept responses that are written by the teacher, an aide, or other students at school.
    - Accept responses that are written by a parent at home. Allow

the parent to do 90 percent of the homework writing. The child, of course, is to do 100 percent of the thinking.

- Require children to write spelling words no more than one time each. (With ten words written just one time each, multiplied by ten times as much effort, an STNR child will still be writing the equivalent of one hundred words.)

- Do *not* use writing as a punishment.
- Grade for content rather than penmanship, or else give a separate grade for each.
- Allow more time for writing tasks.
- Allow children to use a computer.
- Be as pleasant and patient as possible.

Reading and Spelling (Dyslexia)

The problems exhibited by STNR children in the areas of reading and spelling (dyslexia) usually concern reversals, directionality, and sequencing.

Originally the term *dyslexia* referred to a neurological dysfunction that made learning to read extremely difficult. Currently, the term *dyslexia* is used to refer to a variety of problems in numerous areas, from math and spelling to tying shoes. Many of the characteristics of children with dyslexia are identical to the characteristics of children with an immature STNR: reversal of letters and numbers, confusion of right and left, and difficulty with sequencing. While the immature STNR does not directly cause dyslexia, it does interfere with the ease and efficiency of most learning processes. The child with both dyslexia and an immature STNR is doubly handicapped. Now, fortunately, we can "cure" the immature STNR, thereby eliminating many of the problems common to dyslexia.

Reversals
There is much in current educational literature about reversal problems. A reversal refers to a child's tendency to write *b* for *d* or *p* for *q* or *12* for *21* or to read *was* for *saw* or *gril* for *girl*, for example.

Relationship of STNR to Reading

It has been suggested (Blythe 1992) that the symmetrical tonic neck reflex (STNR) helps to complete a sequence of eye training. Bending of the legs as a result of head extension also encourages the infant to "fixate" his eyes at far distance. Bending of the arms in response to flexion of the head (head lowered below the spine line) will automatically bring the child's focus back to near distance, thus training the eyes to adjust from far to near distance and back again. The symmetrical tonic neck reflex brings the vision to near distance, training the readjustment of binocular vision. It remains for the process of creeping on hands and knees to further develop the visual skills the infant has learned so far and to integrate them with information from other senses.

Creeping is one of the most important movement patterns in the prolonged process of teaching the eyes to cross the midline. In addition to looking ahead, babies also learn eye-hand coordination from the movement of the hands. At times, the eyes focus from one hand to another, with the hands acting as moving stimuli. Later on this ability will be essential for being able to read without losing the words at the middle of the line and to visually follow the moving hand when writing. It is through creeping that the vestibular, proprioceptive and visual systems connect to operate together for the first time. Without this integration there can be a poorly developed sense of balance and poor space and depth perception.

The focusing distance and hand-eye coordination skills used in the act of creeping are at the same distance that the child will eventually use for reading and writing. It has been observed (Pavlides 1987) that a high percentage of children with reading difficulties omitted the stages of crawling and creeping in infancy. (Goddard 2002, p. 23)

Theories attempting to explain this phenomenon range from the popular concept of mirror reading (having words actually register backward in the brain) to the more extreme theory that the child has an emotional disturbance and would rather live in the past or the future. (Whew!) We believe, as a result of our clinical experience, that in the case of STNR children, a more probable explanation for these reversals is that a child's "directionality" has not been well established: the child simply goes in the wrong direction. If the child reads from right to left, the word *was* reads as *saw*. Under these circumstances, the reading is accurate, but the direction is wrong. In many cases, children who have been labeled as classic dyslexics may be significantly helped by STNR therapy.

Directionality

Directionality is the awareness of our own right- and left-sidedness in the world around us. Directionality affects the reading of a printed word or number, the choice of a turn at an intersection, the printing of letters, the writing of words, and the ability to find one's way back to the car in the parking lot. All may be achieved by a person with poor directionality, but not quickly or efficiently achieved. A good sense of directionality is essential for *efficient* reading, writing, spelling, math, and motor activities. *Good directionality is essential for efficiency in nearly everything we do.*

Given enough time, the child with poor directionality can usually figure out whether a word is *dab, dad, bad,* or *bab.* However, while the child with poor directionality is figuring it out, the other children have read to the end of the line, and soon they are at the end of the paragraph. The child who was left behind figuring out which direction to go soon begins to wonder whether the other children are smarter. (We must emphasize that poor directionality does not necessarily indicate lesser intelligence. One can be a genius and have poor directionality.)

As we stated in chapter 2, the development of directionality begins with the child's crawling in infancy. As children crawl, they gain awareness of the two sides of their bodies. This awareness of "sidedness" eventually develops into a sense of direction. Children who do not crawl at all, or who crawl for a very short period of time, or who walk very early, or who crawl "funny" will miss out on this essential stage in the development of directionality because they have not crawled properly or long enough to establish the internal awareness of sidedness that develops into directionality. These children will also not mature the STNR, because crawling is essential to the maturation of this reflex. Consequently, these children experience the compound problems of an immature STNR in addition to poor directionality. Learning to read can become very difficult when reversals that are caused by poorly developed directionality combine with the discomfort, shortened attention span, disorganization, increased activity, and physical tension caused by the immature STNR.

Sequencing

Frequently, children with an immature STNR will also have problems with sequencing. This term refers to putting things in their correct order, either according to time or according to place; it is an ability required in spelling, following directions, following the correct steps in math computations, and understanding the concept of time. In school, directionality and sequencing are essential not only in academic courses but also in such classes as home economics, shop, driver education, history, geography . . . the list can go on and on.

Jeff, one of our clients, was a high-school student who came to us for help with driver education. His parents had heard that we were able to help people with directionality and sequencing problems. Jeff's driver-education teacher was concerned because Jeff could not react quickly and with consistent accuracy to such commands as "Go two blocks and turn right," or "Go to the third light and turn left."

Jeff had never crawled as a baby, and he had a history of coordination difficulties. Years of intensive gross-motor programs had brought significant improvement in his coordination, yet he still was bothered by an immature STNR and poorly established directionality and sequencing. The remediation exercises we prescribed not only matured Jeff's STNR, but also helped him develop better directionality and sequencing. (He got his driver's license.)

The development of sequencing begins with the child's crawling in infancy. The movement of first one body part and then another in the proper order for crawling is the beginning of sequencing at its most basic level. We continue to see the importance of sufficient, appropriate crawling. *Crawling* is the common factor in the development of many factors necessary for success in school.

Reading and Spelling Circumventions

The following circumventions will allow STNR children to function better in reading and spelling situations. (Remember: these are circumventions for the STNR, not techniques for teaching reading or spelling.)

- *Allow postural freedom.*
- Keep reading and spelling sessions short, five to fifteen minutes.
- *Do not* use reading or the writing of spelling words as a punishment.
- Allow children to substitute oral book reports or projects for written responses to their reading.
- Allow children to take their spelling tests orally—to the teacher, to an aide, or into a tape recorder.
- Require children to write spelling words no more than one time each. (With ten words written just one time each, multiplied by ten times as much effort, an STNR child will still be writing the equivalent of one hundred words.)
- Allow more time for reading and spelling tasks.
- Refer to the list of general circumventions for problems at school on p. 96.
- Be as pleasant and patient as possible.

Math (Dyscalculia)

Copying math problems from the chalkboard or from a textbook onto a sheet of paper is a task in itself, especially for STNR children. They are exhausted just from the copying, yet they still have the problems to work. Many of these children require much more writing space than the average child. Their work is often sprawled over the page, frequently with "cattywampus" columns running diagonally down the page. The equation 75 plus 21 will not yield 96 if the numbers have been copied in the following manner:

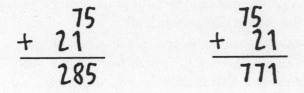

When columns are not kept straight, it is easy to see how a child can "figure right but answer wrong."

Some children try to deal with the interference of the immature STNR by writing very, very small numbers, thereby avoiding excessive arm movement. Unfortunately, their written work is often so cramped and run-together that it is difficult to read. Cramped writing also severely hinders the keeping of accurate columns. These STNR children frequently reverse numbers, so that *21* becomes *12*. We have heard a child mumbling "seventy-one" while writing *17*. This reversal problem is common to children with STNR immaturity and is common in both math and reading.

Sequencing difficulties often loom up for the STNR children in more complicated math problems. Frequently, their errors are not in computation, but in confusion with which step to use next. Many times, incorrect answers are more a product of mistakes in sequencing than mistakes in calculation.

Again, *crawling* is the common denominator (pun intended) in the development of directionality and sequencing—factors necessary for success in math.

Math Circumventions

The following circumventions will help STNR children to do their arithmetic assignments. (Remember: these are circumventions for the STNR, not techniques for teaching arithmetic.)

- *Allow postural freedom.*
- Put fewer problems on a page, allowing room for larger writing.
- Use large graph paper to help children keep columns straight.
- Cut the math paper into quarters, giving one portion at a time. The total assignment will not appear so overwhelming if presented in smaller segments.
- Do not require that children write practice problems or corrected problems more than one time each.
- *Do not* assign arithmetic problems as a punishment.
- Allow others to copy the problems from the book (or chalkboard), so that STNR children can concentrate on working the problems.
- Refer to the list of general circumventions for problems at school on p. 96.
- Be as pleasant and patient as possible.

Art and Music

Standing at an easel in art class is usually a treat for STNR children. The pleasure of art class is reduced for these children when they are required to do their work seated at tables or desks. An immature STNR interferes with the tasks of coloring, cutting, and pasting in the same way that it interferes with writing. Art class activities usually are more fun and easier for STNR children if they are allowed to stand and move around a little. Often, parents have been amazed that their children did not like sitting down and coloring: "We thought all kids loved to color, but Johnny always hated it." Most likely it was the position he hated, not the coloring. Coloring is just like writing. The STNR child who has to sit at a desk is very uncomfortable.

Interestingly enough, some STNR children hate to color, but love to draw. Coloring within the lines is too difficult for their fine-motor (small muscle) skills, and coloring outside the lines is almost a crime in our society. Drawing, however, allows children more freedom with space, reducing fine-motor demands. In drawing, the fine-motor control is of their own choosing. Even when given ample space, some STNR children draw very small and write "teensy." This is another way of trying to control the interfering effects of an immature STNR.

We are frequently told by STNR children that they dislike music class. Usually we discover that it is neither the teacher nor the music that they really dislike. Their most common complaint is, "I have to sit still the whole class time." While the teacher is working with one group, the rest of the children are expected to sit quietly and "sit up straight" until their turn. STNR children cannot sit still comfortably, and their discomfort often generates dislike for the subject.

The reflex also frequently interferes with the coordination necessary for rhythmic tasks. STNR children can often be spotted easily in kindergarten or first grade because they cannot march to even the strongest beat. Teachers often despair of having these children "keep time" in rhythmic activities. (We suspect these children grow up to be rigid or reluctant dance partners.)

Selection of a particular musical instrument can also be a clue. Consider the position required for playing certain instruments. Many STNR children prefer "stand up" instruments (bass violins, trumpets, marimbas) or percussion instruments on which they can release some of their physical tension.

Art and Music Circumventions

The following circumventions will allow STNR children to function better in art and music classes.

- *Allow postural freedom.*
- Modify the situation to help the STNR child get comfortable.
  - Art: Provide high stools or let students stand at easels.
  - Music: Let students stand or lie down while the teacher works with other groups.
    Steer STNR students toward instruments the STNR will not interfere with.
    Let students practice for several shorter sessions, rather than one long session.
- Be as pleasant and patient as possible.

Physical Education

The coordination required for success in physical education is not easily achieved or maintained by children with an immature STNR. They are usually the last ones chosen for a team and the first ones eliminated in activities requiring motor skill. Thus, the very children who most need the opportunity for development of motor coordination end up watching from the sidelines. Some STNR children *prefer* to watch from the sidelines. They may dislike gym because it places them in a situation where their lack of coordination will embarrass them. Sometimes, consciously or unconsciously, these children will try to remove themselves from gym class.

Patty was a charming first-grade child whose parents were concerned about her persistent stomachaches. There was a pattern to these stomachaches; they always occurred on Tuesdays. We have come to expect the *Monday*-morning stomachache or headache, because some children are so reluctant to renew the tensions of school. The Tuesday stomachache was a new one to us.

After much discussion with the parents and teacher, we discovered that the only major difference between Tuesday and the other days was that Tuesday was gym day. Patty was extremely poorly coordinated—awful—in gym. She could not participate successfully with any of the children her age.

No one, not Patty, parents, or teacher, had made the connection between her pitiful performance in gym class, her dislike of gym class, and her weekly stomachaches to avoid gym class. After we were able to help her become better coordinated, her Tuesday-morning stomachaches went away.

Other STNR children may persist in behavior that will eventually exasperate the teacher to the point of removing these children from gym class activities. Many of these children who seem deliberately disruptive in gym class are the victims of the immature STNR. They may be able to perform some motor tasks, but usually not the tasks requested by the gym teacher. A classic example of a motor activity that is popular with STNR children is sliding into gym class on their knees. Many STNR children are proficient at this, but the action is not highly regarded by most gym teachers.

On the other hand, some STNR children like gym class because they have an opportunity to be up and moving. Physical education is frequently their favorite class even though they may perform poorly in many of the activities. Sometimes these children may be able to run fast and even catch well if they are standing still, but they usually have extreme difficulty running and catching at the same time.

Remember that we have stressed that the immature STNR *interferes* with motor coordination rather than totally prohibiting it. Children with an immature STNR have to work extremely hard to learn a simple motor task. With tremendous effort, energy, and desire, STNR children may be able to learn almost any motor task appropriate to their ages. Although they may eventually even do rather well, they will probably have more bruises, cuts, and scrapes than the average child. Comments such as "awkward," "clumsy," and "trips over his own feet" are frequent descriptions of the majority of these children. However, while the interference by the STNR can be very obvious, it also may be very subtle.

STNR children can become skilled in almost any motor task,
but only at the expense of unbelievable time, effort, and energy.

Physical Education Circumventions
The following circumventions will allow STNR children to function better in physical education classes. Note: Because STNR children will usually be the last ones chosen for teams, *teachers* should always *assign* teams rather than having student captains choose sides. Do not tolerate negative comments or moaning when children are assigned to teams.

- Play games in which children are not quickly eliminated due to poor performances.

- Adapt the rules of games so that no one is eliminated.
  - Put time limits on teams, rather than removing players from the game.
  - Keep score, rather than eliminating players from the game (e.g., in musical chairs, put the name of the child who is "out" on the board, but allow the player to stay in the game).
  - Allow players to earn their way back into the game (e.g., in dodge ball, a player who is hit can become active again if a teammate catches the ball or if the team members avoid being hit three times in a row).
- Be as pleasant and patient as possible.

Accelerated and Enrichment Classes

The immature reflex does not respect intelligence. It can and does occur in children who span the entire range of intelligence, from the mentally deficient, to average, to above average, to gifted. While this reflex can be very interfering for people at all levels of intelligence, it can be particularly exasperating for gifted children.

Remember: the STNR remains immature regardless of intellectual superiority unless there is sufficient and proper crawling.

Many of the gifted STNR children who have come to our clinic exhibit the following characteristics:

- They walked early, crawling for only a short time.
- They were classified as behavior problems because of their resistance to academic demands.
- Many had not been identified as gifted because of their poor performance academically.
- They were classified as underachievers because of their resistance to the school's demand to put everything in writing.

Some gifted STNR children do well in school, at least for a while, because of their superior verbal abilities. Some parents and teachers just laugh off the illegible writing of these children, saying they are all going to grow up to be doctors. However, an immature STNR can cause not only illegibility, but also a strong resistance to writing.

Consider the story of Ted, a gifted reader. When he was in the second grade, he was reading at the sixth-grade level. We were very surprised, therefore, to hear from his fourth-grade teacher that Ted was failing reading. We couldn't imagine how that was possible. Then the teacher said, "He just refuses to write his book reports." Of course, for us, the word *write* set off alarms. The crawling test for immature STNR interference indicated that the reflex was significantly interfering with Ted's writing ease, and he just refused to do what was uncomfortable and inefficient for him.

For this resistance to writing, STNR children with average intelligence are called "lazy." Gifted STNR children are called "bored." Although parents do not like to have their children called lazy, some parents seem proud to have their children called bored. "Boredom" seems to suggest intellectual superiority. We strongly believe that most of these so-called "bored" gifted students are not intellectually bored by the concepts of the material. Instead, they are bored by the hassle of spending many hours trying to *write* what they grasped intellectually in a few minutes.

We believe that many gifted STNR children drop out because the immature STNR makes their written work so laborious for them. "Many gifted and talented students drop out of school at rates far exceeding the rates of dropouts for their nongifted peers." (Ryan and Cooper 1995) What a waste of natural resources!

Circumventions for Accelerated and Enrichment Classes

The following circumventions will allow gifted STNR children to be more comfortable and efficient in meeting greater academic demands.

- Do not double or triple or quadruple the STNR children's writing assignments in a misguided attempt to challenge them intellectually.

- Refer to the list of general circumventions for problems at school on this page.
- Be as pleasant and patient as possible.

General Circumventions in School

Throughout this chapter, we discuss numerous circumventions specific to various academic situations. The more general circumventions presented below will allow STNR children to function more efficiently and more comfortably in school.

- Allow postural freedom. Standing up, or lying on the floor, or sitting on their legs will probably be more comfortable for STNR children than sitting at a desk in the "proper sitting position." STNR children will accomplish more work if they are more comfortable. (Do not allow postures that are potentially dangerous.) Do not require the child to sit unless it is absolutely necessary, which is actually rare. Think about it.
- Require less writing.
  - Reduce all written work to the barest minimum. If an assignment is mainly concerned with a one-word answer, let the children write the one word rather than having to copy an entire sentence.
  - Give clear, well-reproduced duplicated sheets of math problems or let another student copy the problems from the book rather than making the STNR children do all of that writing before even getting around to working the problem.
  - Allow STNR children to underline or circle answers rather than writing them out.
  - Accept single-word answers rather than complete sentences.
  - For work done in school, accept student responses that are written by the teacher, an aide, or by other students.

- For work done at home, accept student responses written by a parent. (Most parents are conscientious about schoolwork and will not cheat for their children.)
- Instead of writing responses, allow children to give oral responses to the teacher, to an aide, or into a tape recorder.

- Give shorter writing assignments. Several shorter assignments are preferable to one long assignment. A child who has a history of failure will be reluctant to attempt an assignment that seems very long. Frequently the teacher can successfully encourage the child to do the assignment by breaking it up into several shorter assignments, sometimes literally cutting the page of problems into fourths and giving the child a fourth of a page at a time.

- Allow more time for writing tasks.

- Allow STNR children to use a computer for assignments. Even the hunt-and-peck method can be easier and more efficient for these children to perform than writing, and will almost certainly be more legible. Computers can significantly facilitate writing for STNR children. The children may need help with proofreading.

- Allow chalkboard work as an alternative to paperwork (especially for the teaching of handwriting itself).

- Grade for content rather than for quality of penmanship, or give a separate grade for each.

- Provide sufficient working space on worksheets and make certain that the worksheet is clear. Although most children can do better work if the worksheet is clearly legible and there is ample space for writing their answers, these criteria are essential for children with motor difficulties, perceptual difficulties, or both. Though this may seem to be a minor point, it can sometimes make the difference between a child's willingness or unwillingness to attempt a task.

- *Do not* assign arithmetic problems or any writing assignment as a punishment.

- Be as patient and pleasant as possible. We cannot stress this enough.

Teachers should remember that it will not always be easy to be as patient and pleasant as possible, but we feel it will always be rewarding to you and to your students.

Please note that we *are not* asking for lessened responsibilities for STNR students. We are asking for modifications to help these students learn more easily and to demonstrate more easily what they really know. Parents should remember that any circumvention requires extra time and effort from already busy teachers.

You must learn to be detectives, to look for clues, *to analyze the nature of the task*. The effect of the STNR is more subtle than obvious. For example, a child with both arms stuck straight out in casts would not be expected to do written homework or to eat neatly at the table. Having both arms in casts is a rather obvious interference. Even most psychologists would consider the casts the primary source of interference, though some, we are certain, would suggest that the child had deliberately broken both arms as a means of defiance or to avoid doing homework. Perhaps the child could "try a little harder" and learn to write with his toes. The effect of an immature STNR is not so obvious as having casts on both arms, but, in the long run, nearly as interfering. An immature STNR can create significant interference with academic achievement.

If your child is having problems with schoolwork, consider that the major problem may be an immature STNR.

Read on to discover how the immature STNR can cause problems with sports.

6. Sports Problems

How does the immature STNR interfere with sports? An immature STNR can be directly responsible for poor motor coordination (resulting in clumsiness or awkwardness). Poor coordination usually contributes to poor performance in athletics. Poor performance usually limits participation. Limited participation, in turn, prolongs poor performance. It becomes a vicious cycle.

In American society, participation in sports is almost mandatory for boys. Society's demands are essentially met if a boy participates in sports, even if he doesn't excel in them. Whether that is the way it should be or not, that is the way it is. While the social demand for participation in sports is not yet so strong for girls, support and praise are increasing for girls who are successful in sports.

An immature STNR usually affects children's athletic performance in one of two ways. Generally, these children do very poorly in most sports. However, some STNR children may do fairly well in certain sports. Either they work ten times harder than other children to achieve some success, or the immature STNR does not interfere with the body position required for success in that particular sport.

Your child may seem well coordinated, but only in certain sports. The interference of the reflex can be very tricky. The immature reflex causes the top half of the body to want to do the opposite from the bottom half. It is very difficult for STNR children to have their bodies either all straight or all bent at the same time.

For example, it is very difficult for STNR children to run and catch at the same time. They have trouble looking up in the air and following the ball without stumbling or falling to the ground. Remember, as the neck and arms straighten, the immature STNR makes the knees want to bend. There really are no circumventions for STNR children in sports. The most helpful approach is to mature the reflex through the STNR crawling exercises. The next most helpful approach is to recognize the symptoms of the immature reflex and steer the child into specific sports and positions that will not be negatively affected by an immature STNR. Let us consider how the reflex can interfere with specific sports.

Baseball

The ordinary tasks of catching and throwing do not come easily for STNR children. They must labor to *barely acquire* simple skills while other children are refining and improving the same skills.

One of our young clients was brought to us by a very determined mother—and a very reluctant father. (You could almost see the heel marks in the carpet where the mother had dragged the father down the hall and into our clinic.) The father's first words were, "I don't see how she can say David has a coordination problem. He's won the player-of-the-year award in Little League for three years in a row."

The father went on to explain that David had won this award as an outfielder. This was unusual because the Little League coaches generally put the worst players in the outfield to keep them out of the way, though coaches will occasionally put one good player in the outfield to chase the ball so that every hit does not become a home run. This particular boy was obviously one of those better outfielders, which amazed us, because our reflex test indicated that he had the immature STNR at a very interfering level.

We told the parents that we would explain the usual effects of the reflex, and see whether the description applied at all to their son. About halfway through our explanation, the father looked very surprised and said, "Well, that explains it."

We asked, "Explains what?"

"That explains why he catches the way he does," the father answered.

Intrigued, we asked how David caught. Since David had an immature STNR, when he raised his head and straightened his arms to catch a fly ball, his legs would want to bend. And that's exactly what happened. To control the effects of the reflex, David dropped to the ground on his knees every time he made a catch, realizing that he was more stable that way, but not knowing why. The father told us that they had originally thought David was "hot dogging," or showing off. They had tried to get him to catch in a more traditional way, but he was so successful in catching his own way that they had decided not to mess with his success.

David's catching style was evidently successful enough for Little League. At higher levels of competition, however, having to get up from a kneeling position every time before relaying the ball could cost valuable seconds, and not many players are efficient at throwing from their knees.

On another occasion, we were watching Richard, a nine-year-old, throwing a ball to his mother. He threw with his right hand and appropriately stepped forward with his left foot. Since he had been brought to us because of poor coordination, we were surprised at how well he threw the ball.

His father sighed and said, "You'll never know how long we've worked on proper throwing." He told us that they had spent hours showing and telling their son, "You step with your left foot; you throw with your right hand." A skill that usually develops quickly and easily for most children had taken hours of time, effort, and energy for Richard and his parents.

Batting is another important facet of baseball. Many young children learning to bat stand relatively upright, with their arms bent.

This position is very comfortable for a child with an immature STNR. However, while the legs are straight, STNR children must "explode" their arm muscles in order to straighten their arms and hit the ball. If these children hit the ball, they usually hit it a long way. If they miss, they usually spin completely around. They cannot "check" their swings: it's really difficult to stop an explosion. These children will rarely be seen in a crouched batter's position with their arms and legs bent at the same time, although they may like to crouch and keep their arms straight out.

Baseball provides a classic example of a position that allows the interference of the STNR to be avoided or bypassed. For example, the usual catcher's position may be naturally easier for STNR children since they can bend their knees and extend their arms very comfortably. Nevertheless, the reflex usually interferes with many other motor requirements of baseball.

Basketball

Dribbling a basketball is a very sophisticated motor activity. Dribbling a ball and running at the same time are even more complex. Many STNR children have *great difficulty* dribbling a basketball. Most STNR children have *extreme* difficulty trying to dribble the ball and run. It is almost *impossible* for STNR children to run, dribble, and control the ball when another player is trying to take it away.

Some STNR children who aren't good ball handlers may, nevertheless, become good shooters. It is extremely difficult for STNR children to have their bodies all bent at the same time; therefore, most of them prefer to stop and get set before shooting, rather than running and jumping and shooting. While the set shot may be as accurate, the jump shot is more popular in today's fast game. It must be very frustrating to the coaches—and to these STNR players—to try to add an accurate jump shot to their basketball repertoire. We suspect many a coach wonders how a player can be so proficient in one aspect of a sport and so poor in another. (Now you know.)

Volleyball

Volleyball, like basketball, is a sport that attracts girls as well as boys. We have been interested in watching the women's volleyball team at our university. We can tell within minutes which team members have STNR involvement: they lose their balance more often; they frequently have more injuries; they usually have more bruises.

However, interestingly enough, STNR players often have a very strong "spike." (A spike is a sharp, hard, downward slam of the ball.) When a player with an immature STNR leaps into the air with bent legs, assuming the arms are bent, there is an STNR "explosion" of muscle in order to straighten the arms. Therefore, in spite of the generally interfering influence of the STNR, some volleyball players can take advantage of this explosive force made available to them. Nevertheless, even though this "explosion" can contribute to a very effective spike, the STNR interferes with overall coordination. STNR players frequently fall to the floor, eliminating themselves from further participation, at least for a few seconds; of course, if the spike is good enough, that play may already be over.

Football

As we saw in baseball, basketball, and volleyball, the contradiction of motor coordination and "discombobulation" in the same person can be seen in many sports. STNR children frequently think we are psychic because we can tell them what positions they play in different sports.

In football, STNR players are rarely the quarterbacks, who run and throw, or the wide receivers, who run and catch. We have seen a few receivers who managed to succeed although they were, we suspect, bothered by the STNR: they either fell down as they caught the ball, or they caught it very close to the ground and ran with their knees significantly bent. Of course, it is difficult to run fast when one is all bent over. Many young athletes with the STNR bothering them become quite adept at forcefully propelling their entire bodies forward. They make fine tackles and guards, but seldom excel as receivers or backs. With the STNR at an interfering level, coordinated interaction of the upper and lower limbs is very difficult to achieve and maintain.

Swimming

Some parents of children brought to our clinic tell us that their children are fine swimmers. We usually find that these children are either strong kickers, with their arms doing a kind of dog paddle, or they are strong arm strokers, with their legs barely fluttering. While these children may be "strong" swimmers, they are rarely efficient or proficient swimmers in the freestyle.

Most STNR children have great difficulty succeeding in progressive stages of swimming programs. Many parents tell us that their children never pass the "guppy" or "tadpole" levels. Everyone becomes so frustrated that swimming lessons are often discontinued.

Usually, STNR children prefer to swim underwater. They have enough trouble trying to coordinate their arms and legs without also having to coordinate their breathing. Swimming underwater, they just hold their breath.

The very nature of swimming provides opportunities to bypass or avoid the interference of the reflex by assuming comfortable body positions. STNR children would probably learn to swim more easily and quickly if their instructors would start them with the butterfly or breaststroke rather than the freestyle. In the breaststroke and the butterfly, the arms are straight or must straighten while the legs are bent to kick. In the freestyle, too many parts of the body (the neck, the arms, and the legs) have to bend or turn at the same time.

John was a former student of ours who displayed hyperactive behaviors. He had trouble maintaining attention; he would not sit still; he talked constantly; and he avoided writing (unless he was allowed to lie on the window ledge). John did not distinguish himself academically in high school. Even though he had above-average intelligence, he performed academically just well enough to remain on the swim team. Considering his behavioral characteristics, we now strongly suspect that John was suffering from an immature STNR. How, then, was he able to be a medalist on the high-school swim team?

His best stroke was the butterfly, and his next best was the breaststroke. He was so poor at the freestyle that he was never selected as a member of the relay team, yet he won medal after medal in the butterfly and breaststroke events.

Occasionally, certain aspects of certain sports may actually be facilitated or assisted, or at least not hindered, by the presence of an immature STNR. Remember, however, that overall coordination is always better with the reflex at a mature level.

Wrestling

Many of the boys we see in our clinic are wrestlers. Frequently, they had not successfully participated in any sport until wrestling became available to them. One young boy walked in and looked at the chalkboard, where we had drawn the basic position of the STNR (figure 6.1),

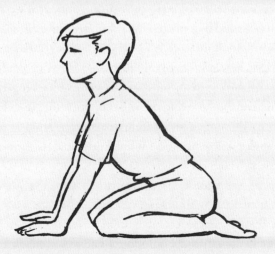

FIGURE 6.1. **The Cat Sit Position**

"That's one of our wrestling positions," he said. "Why are you drawing pictures about wrestling?"

We began to analyze some of the actions of wrestling: in order to move out of the cat sit position, a wrestler with an immature STNR must "explode" forward. This explosion provides an advantage over the opponent and helps compensate for general deficiency in coordination. Remember, however, that overall coordination is always better with the reflex at a mature level.

Hockey

Another sport, another story:

A mother brought her seven-year-old son to us. After hearing about the reflex, she said, "That certainly describes Andy, although it sounds even more like his older brother. But he's a professional hockey player."

We said, "Are you sure?"

She replied, "I guess I know what my son does for a living, and he is a professional hockey player."

We all laughed as we assured her that we were not really questioning her knowledge of her son's profession, but we were surprised that he could be a professional hockey player if he displayed symptoms of an immature STNR. We asked ourselves how—assuming that he *did* have an immature STNR—he would be able to skate with his head up and then down, watching the puck, bending his arms as he swings the hockey stick, bending his legs to skate, and do all of this well enough to earn a living at it. Finally we thought to ask his mother, "What position does he play?"

She replied, "He's the goalie."

Of course; we should have known. Picture the goalie as he squats on bent legs, with arms extended. The reflex does not interfere with such a position. It is even possible that if a hockey goalie had an immature STNR the reflex would make him more comfortable for extended periods of time in that position. (We are certainly not implying that all goalies have an immature STNR. However, his mother's description definitely suggested that this particular goalie did have an immature STNR.)

Soccer

Every day we thank God for soccer because it provides opportunities for athletic success for many STNR children. Remember, children with an immature STNR have trouble coordinating the top and bottom parts of their bodies. Coordinating their arms with their legs is very difficult for them. In soccer, the rules prohibit any player (except the goalie) from using arms and hands, thereby reducing the coordination requirements for STNR players.

Soccer is mostly a running and kicking sport. Even though running is always more efficient with good arm interaction, it can be accomplished, even fairly effectively, with limited interaction of the arms. What a perfect sport soccer is for STNR children.

Skiing

Skiing is another activity that primarily involves the legs. The bent-leg position required for downhill skiing is basically comfortable for STNR children, if nothing is required of their arms at the same time. Frequently, small children beginning to ski do not use poles, but learn to navigate totally with their legs. Once leg control is mastered, poles are added. Skiers with an immature STNR can be easily spotted on the slopes by the awkward or rigid manner in which they hold their ski poles. Nevertheless, they may become proficient enough to enjoy recreational skiing.

Golf and Tennis

If people play golf and tennis properly, their knees are bent and their arms are straight. Golf and tennis are "naturals" for individuals with STNR immaturity although STNR golfers may have trouble keeping their heads down while their arms are extended. Even though their movements may not be fluid or graceful, they may hit the ball fairly well. (One friend described her husband as looking like a robot when he played golf and tennis although he was relatively successful.) With proper instruction, children and adults with STNR involvement may perform well and enjoy golf and tennis.

Summary

A child with STNR immaturity may learn most motor skills, but only with incredible effort and intense desire. What we are stressing is that these children have to work harder to develop certain motor skills than children without the STNR immaturity.

Parents, teachers, and coaches need to pay attention to the *process* as well as the *product*. *How* something is accomplished is at least as important as *what* is accomplished. Most children do not have to spend days and weeks learning what appear to be relatively easy skills. In cases where a child seems to display an enduring lack of motivation, inattention, lack of cooperation, disorganization, and lack of effort, *we urge you to consider the possibility of STNR interference.*

As you can see from the case histories we have described throughout this book, recognizing the interference of the STNR can be tricky. You must learn to be detectives, to look for clues, *to analyze the nature of the task.* The STNR does not interfere with every activity, only with certain ones. In a way, identifying an STNR child would be easier if the reflex interfered with every activity. However, STNR involvement is inhibitive—selectively interfering—rather than prohibitive—totally blocking the activity. Through diligence, determination, and drive (time, effort, and energy), or through selection of certain body positions easier for them, some STNR children may become surprisingly successful in various sports. This is why we say the STNR is "tricky": *STNR children who spend the extra time, effort, and energy, or who choose certain positions, may appear well coordinated, when in fact they are not.*

Remember: *we are not saying* that the STNR is prohibitive. STNR children may seem very well coordinated if they excel in certain sports or physical activities. Their level of excellence may come from tremendous effort or from the selection of a sport that "bypasses" the STNR interference. *We are saying* that you should be careful not to assume that a child is truly well coordinated because of success in a given sport or aspect of a specific sport. *Life in general is difficult for STNR children, even if they manage to do well in sports.*

If your child is having problems with sports, consider that the major problem may be an immature STNR.

Read on to discover how the immature STNR can cause problems at home.

7.　Problems at Home

How does the immature STNR cause problems at home? What is it like living with STNR children? Is it fun? Is it fun to have dinner, watch television, or try to read the paper next to a child in constant motion? Is it fun to try to help STNR children with their homework? Usually, it is not much fun at all. The therapy described in Part Three of this book can change that situation, but in the meantime the circumventions in this chapter can make life much more pleasant for parent and child.

Mealtime

In our society as it is today, dinner is one of the few occasions when a family is together. It should be a pleasant time. However, for families with STNR children, mealtime can be considerably less than pleasant. Remember Billy, whose home situation we described in chapter 3? Negative comments were all he heard at the dinner table:

"Billy, sit down."
"Billy, quit kicking your sister."
"Billy, don't eat so fast."
"Billy, get off your foot and sit on your chair."

"Billy, you almost knocked your milk over again."
"Billy, would you PLEASE sit still?"

Under those conditions, eating a meal could not be very pleasant for Billy or for anyone else at the table. Who would look forward to mealtime with the family? What do you think it does for a child's self-esteem to have his name always followed by something negative? (A child we know thought his name was "Johnny No" because that's all he ever heard.)

Please understand that we are not being critical of parents. Enjoying a meal and instilling some manners in a child are difficult when the child is all over the chair and table. The behavior of STNR children may not be "bad," but it is often irritating. Being around them for a long period of time without being critical of their behavior is difficult, especially when one does not understand why they act the way they do.

We think that a major reason for this undesirable dinner table behavior is an immature STNR. What do many families emphasize at the dinner table? . . . Sitting down and sitting still. These tasks are made more difficult for STNR children because they must constantly be bending their arms while eating. This creates a tension and discomfort similar to that produced by sitting and writing at school. Many tasks required of children at home are similar to those required of them at school, but the similarities may not be easily recognized. Identifying the real problem is essential before appropriate remediation can be selected.

Mealtime Circumventions

The following circumventions will help the STNR child and the entire family enjoy mealtime more:

- *Allow postural freedom.* The STNR child may be more comfortable standing at the table or at the kitchen counter or sitting on one or both legs and may need to get up from the table occasionally. We are not in favor of unsafe positions, such as tipping the chair back or sitting on the back of the chair.
- Provide helpful seating arrangements. Put the STNR child at the

end of the table, for example, where there is more room to move without disturbing others. At least, do not crowd the STNR child in the middle.

- Be as pleasant and patient as possible.

Many benefits are gained when these circumventions are put into effect. Mealtime is generally more pleasant, with less fussing, less wiggling, less arguing and complaining, and fewer spills. Often, there is an improvement in the STNR child's eating habits, and certainly in self-esteem.

Homework

Consider homework. How many parents require their children to sit at a desk or table to do their homework? Parents frequently ask, "Surely children will do their homework better if they are sitting up straight, won't they? That's how they do it at school." And so, many loving parents buy desks for their children in an effort to help them develop good study habits. Then these parents are frustrated and perplexed when their children prefer to lie on the floor to do their homework.

One mother told us that she helped her twelve-year-old son, Tom, study social studies every night. This mother and son seemed to have a very good relationship, and they tried to make each session a pleasant one. Tom would diligently read his social studies by himself for ten to fifteen minutes, lying on the floor. When his mother came in to quiz him on his reading, she would say, "You can't really study lying on the floor." She would make Tom get up and sit at a table. The fact that he *had been studying* was completely missed. At the table, mother and son studied together fairly well for five or ten minutes, but then study conditions and patience progressively deteriorated, with the study session usually ending in a shouting match.

Many psychologists would interpret this as a classic parent/child confrontation. Many would say that the son was being difficult because he did not get his own way. What do you think we would say? Yes . . . immature STNR. The immature STNR was interfering with the child's ability to sit still and upright during the second part of the study session. We must all learn to consider the probability of a physical cause before jumping to the always available, ever-ready psychological interpretations!

The interference of an immature STNR is often the underlying cause for the persistent homework problem: leaving the homework at school. These STNR children have struggled so hard all day to sit still and write that they can't face an additional entire evening of the same torture. An immature STNR is often the main reason why children won't bring home their homework in the first place, procrastinate starting their work even if they do bring it home, will write down any answer just to get the assignment finished, and refuse to check their papers for fear of having to do them again.

Homework Circumventions

The following circumventions will help the STNR child study and complete homework assignments more easily:

- *Allow postural freedom.* The STNR child may be more comfortable sitting in an unconventional posture, standing, lying down or upside down, and getting up from the table or desk occasionally.
- Keep study sessions short. Limit them to ten or fifteen minutes, with a break before the next session.
- Provide pencil "cushions." (These are small rubber or soft plastic sleeves that fit over the pencil to relax the child's "death grip" on the pencil. There are several types on the market.)
- Do 90 percent of the writing for the child. The child should do 100 percent of the thinking. Parents can do the writing.
- Be as pleasant and patient as possible.

Benefits gained from using these circumventions usually include less hassle in doing homework, less fatigue, better use of time, and improved self-esteem.

After-School Fatigue or Overactivity

Another clue to the presence of an immature STNR is exhibited by children who come home from school totally fatigued. Having worked ten times as hard as their classmates all day long, they are not just understandably tired, but really exhausted. They flop onto the couch or take a nap when most children, after a brief rest, are ready to go again. Their fatigue plays a major role in their resistance to doing their homework.

However, remember that the reflex is tricky. In some children, instead of producing after-school fatigue, the reflex produces the opposite reaction. These children, after holding in the physical tension from the reflex all day, almost explode when they get home. They can be really "hyped up."

We were told about one youngster who would burst through the front door, drop his books, race out the back door, and run non-stop for fifteen or twenty minutes. In bad weather he headed for the basement and ran figure eight's around the basement poles. Interestingly, no excessive activity level had been reported by the school. The parents couldn't believe that he was relatively quiet at school; the teacher could not believe that he was so active at home.

After-School Circumventions

The following circumventions will help the STNR child cope with after-school fatigue or overactivity:

- Give a break from school of at least thirty to sixty minutes so that the child can either rest or run off pent-up tension. STNR children need time off before they start their homework.
- Provide a nutritious snack to help maintain the child's energy at the proper level.
- Be as pleasant and patient as possible.

Benefits gained usually include having a more relaxed child who is less resistant to starting homework.

Music Lessons

Another trouble spot on the home front may be music lessons that require sitting in a confined position. STNR children may willingly practice for fifteen minutes twice a day, but will balk at having to practice for thirty minutes straight. Many parents have reported dramatic improvement in their children's attitudes and level of performance when they were allowed to practice their music for several ten- or fifteen-minute sessions, rather than a single long practice session. These children frequently are willing to work (even ten times as hard) for short sessions, but they just cannot maintain the effort over a longer period of time.

Music Practice Circumventions

The following circumventions will help the STNR child during music lessons and practice sessions:

- *Allow postural freedom.* The STNR child may be more comfortable standing (even at the piano) or sitting on one or both legs.
- Schedule several *short* practice sessions of ten to fifteen minutes instead of one long session.
- Be as pleasant and patient as possible.

Benefits gained usually include sustained interest in music and less fuss about practicing.

Familiy Recreation, Games, and Television

Family recreation and games should be fun. Often it is just the opposite for STNR children. Many games require the same skills needed in schoolwork and sports, and STNR children have not perfected these skills. Consequently, they cannot successfully participate in the activities at family picnics and parties.

Another potential disaster area at home is in front of the TV (not to mention what's *on* TV). Some children, believe it or not, can sit still and watch TV quietly, but STNR children are usually on the move when not allowed to assume positions that are comfortable for them. However, given freedom of posture, even STNR children can watch TV relatively quietly.

One mother, distressed by the school's labeling her child as hyper-active, insisted, "He will watch TV by the hour without moving." When we asked her to describe his sitting position while he watched television, she exclaimed, "Oh, he doesn't sit! He lies on the floor in front of the TV with his chin in his hands, or sometimes he will stretch out in the reclining chair." As we smiled at her description, a look of new understanding crossed her face. "Oh, my," she said, "but he has to sit up straight at school, doesn't he?" A seeming dis-crepancy between his activity level at school and at home was now explained.

Family Recreation, Games, and Television Circumventions

The following circumventions will help the STNR child during recreational activities:

- *Allow postural freedom.* The STNR child may be more comfort-able in a beanbag chair or a reclining chair, lying on the floor, standing, or sitting in a variety of positions.
- Encourage STNR children to participate in a variety of activi-ties. You *must* start at a level where they can succeed if you want them to participate.
- Encourage cooperative games rather than emphasizing competi-tive games. In tennis or Ping-Pong, for example, the object of the game could be to keep the ball in play rather than to win the point.
- Refer to the list of general circumventions for problems at home on page 117.
- Be as pleasant and patient as possible.

General Circumventions at Home

Throughout this chapter, we discuss numerous circumventions specific to various home situations. The more general circumventions presented below will allow STNR children to function more comfortably in a wide range of home situations.

- Allow postural freedom. Remember that the STNR child is more comfortable standing or lying down than sitting up straight, and that many of the positions that seem uncomfortable or sloppy to you may actually be comfortable for them. STNR children who have been sitting for a while need to get up and change position to relieve the tension that the reflex causes. Please note that we are not in favor of unsafe positions, such as sitting with a chair tipped back on its rear legs or sitting on the back of a chair. Do not require the child to sit unless it is absolutely necessary, which is actually rare. Think about it.
- Keep activities short or provide breaks.
- Make sure that the child has time to rest before a difficult activity. Remember that fighting the effects of the reflex can leave a child tense and exhausted.
- Provide a nutritious snack to help maintain the child's energy at the proper level.
- Provide helpful seating arrangements. Seat the STNR child where there is room to move, to shift position, without disturbing others.
- Be as pleasant and patient as possible. We cannot stress this enough.

Benefits gained usually include an increase in participation in family activities, along with enjoyment of these activities. Successful and pleasant participation almost certainly leads to improved self-esteem.

If your child is having problems with various home situations, consider that the major problem may be an immature STNR.

Read on to discover how the immature STNR can cause problems in public settings.

8. Problems in Public Settings

How does the immature STNR cause problems outside the school or home, in the wider community? The grief that STNR children experience and cause at home is intensified when they go out in public. Generally speaking, parents and society expect children to display better behavior in public than is required of them at home. STNR children can be disruptive because of the discomfort that the immature reflex causes them. Because of the effects of the STNR on their behavior in public, children are often accused of being poorly disciplined when, in fact, they are just extremely uncomfortable.

The circumventions described in this chapter can make the child more comfortable in public situations—which, in turn, will make the child more welcome in those situations.

Traveling

Traveling with STNR children can be stressful for all concerned. STNR children are generally very uncomfortable and become fretful and fatigued from trying to sit in a confined area, such as a car or an airplane. One family told us that their small car always caused a sensation at stoplights because their seven-year-old would rock back and forth, releasing the tension of his immature STNR and making the entire car shake. The shaking car may have been amusing to the onlookers, but it was probably no fun for the occupants.

Traveling Circumventions

The following circumventions will lead to more pleasant and relaxing times while traveling and after arriving at the destination:

- *Allow postural freedom,* as much as the rules of safety allow.
- Provide as much room as possible, choosing a station wagon or van rather than a small car.
- Take short breaks at least once an hour to allow the child to get out of the car and stretch.
- Refer to the list of general circumventions for public situations on page 125.
- Be as pleasant and patient as possible.

Restaurants

STNR children who have trouble sitting still at the dinner table at home will have even more trouble trying to sit "extra straight" and "extra still" in public restaurants. Because of their inability to meet these "extra" demands, their behavior is often considered worse in public than it is at home.

Restaurant Circumventions

The following circumventions will make dining out with STNR children more pleasant and may even improve digestion:

- *Allow postural freedom.* In a casual restaurant, the STNR child is likely to be more comfortable standing at a counter, sitting on one or both legs, or getting up from the table occasionally, rather than sitting straight and still. We are not in favor of unsafe positions, such as tipping the chair back or sitting on the back of the chair.
- Choose a helpful seating arrangement. Request a corner table, so that standing or moving around a little will not disturb other

people, or put the STNR child at the end of the table, where there is more room to move without disturbing others. Avoid crowding the STNR child between other diners.

- Choose a casual restaurant rather than a formal one, so that there will be less likelihood of the STNR child's disturbing other diners.
- Try not to be concerned about the opinions of other people so long as your child is not loud and remains close to your table. If you find the circumventions or the child's behavior too distasteful, don't eat out.
- Refer to the list of general circumventions for public situations on pages 126–27.
- Be as pleasant and patient as possible.

Religious Services

Often it is easy to spot STNR children in churches, synagogues, and other places of worship. They are uncommonly antsy throughout the services: crawling under the pew, climbing all over the pew, squirming, and shuffling books and papers. Parents often become extremely exasperated when their children "act out" in front of everyone during the service. (Catholic parents have jokingly told us that worship services may be a little easier for Catholic STNR children, since they are not only allowed, but expected, to get up and down a lot.)

One of our young clients, Betsy, had a double "problem": she had an immature STNR, *and* her father was the minister. Her mother had been especially insistent that Betsy sit quietly during her father's sermons. After ten minutes of diligent effort to sit still, Betsy would begin to wiggle. Her mother would then take Betsy outside, shake her, and ask, "Why can't you sit still?" Most services ended with both mother and daughter in tears.

Religious Services Circumventions

The following circumventions will help the STNR child attend religious services more comfortably, with less disruption and greater opportunity for spiritual meditation:

- *Allow postural freedom.* Take a seat in a back row and let the child stand up. Let a small child lie down in the pew.
- Try to find a location where the STNR child can attend to the service without disrupting others: for example a vestibule, a "crying room," or an adjoining chapel.
- Refer to the list of general circumventions for public situations on pages 126–27.
- Be as pleasant and patient as possible.

The Doctor's Office

A typical hour's wait in a doctor's office is difficult for anyone, but waiting is especially difficult for STNR children. Coloring or dot-to-dotting or sitting to read is not easy for these children. Consequently, they tend to walk or climb or run around waiting rooms. Parents and children learn to dread these waiting-room sessions. The other patients and the receptionists, with no knowledge of the STNR problem, often consider STNR children undisciplined, hyperactive, or both.

Visits to the eye doctor can be doubly stressful for STNR children. Not only are they expected to sit still in the waiting room, but they are expected to sit still during the examination. Unfortunately, excessive wiggling and the physical tension caused by the need to wiggle might distort the results of the eye examination.

On the other hand, STNR children have found that certain aspects of visits with dentists have become less stressful with the advent of the reclining chair. At least these children do not have to sit upright for an extended period of time without moving a muscle.

Doctor's Office Circumventions

The following circumventions will lead to less commotion and frustration in the waiting room and more pleasant and accurate examinations:

- *Allow postural freedom.* Allow the child to stand during physical and eye examinations.

- If possible, make yours the first appointment for the morning or afternoon, in order to avoid as much waiting as possible.
- Take quiet games, toys, or activities along with you for the child to play with while waiting.
- Try not to worry about what other people think so long as your child is not being significantly disruptive.
- Be as pleasant and patient as possible.

Barbershops and Beauty Salons

By now you should realize why STNR children have great difficulty when they get their hair cut or styled: they are expected to sit and wait until their turn comes, and they are expected to sit still while getting their hair styled. This extended, motionless sitting is not easy for average children. It is terribly difficult for STNR children.

Barbershop and Beauty Salon Circumventions

The following circumventions will lead to less commotion and frustration while waiting and, probably, better hairdos.

- *Allow postural freedom.* While waiting, an STNR child will be more comfortable sitting on his or her legs or sitting with the legs stretched out. During hair-cutting, the child is likely to be more comfortable standing than sitting.
- If possible, make yours the first appointment in the morning or afternoon, in order to avoid as much waiting as possible.
- Take quiet games, toys, or activities along with you for the child to play with while waiting.
- Be as pleasant and patient as possible.

Spectator Events

Events that should be "just for fun," such as circuses, ice skating revues, movies, plays, concerts, and sports contests, often become anything but fun for STNR children and their families. In today's world, unfortunately, family togetherness is becoming a rare commodity. For the STNR family, *pleasant* family togetherness is even more rare. How tragic for the family when the potential for excitement and joy from a family activity turns into frustration and exasperation because the STNR child cannot sit still! Too many family outings are reduced to, "If you can't sit still, we'll just go home. We'll never take you out again!"

Spectator Event Circumventions

The following circumventions will lead to less commotion and frustration and more fun:

- *Allow postural freedom.* Get aisle seats so that the child can take a break without disturbing the entire row. Look for seats, such as those in the front row of a movie theater, that allow the child to stretch his or her legs without making the extended legs a safety hazard. Select theaters that provide more leg room, e.g., those with stadium seating.
- Select short events or take a break in the middle, even if it means missing a small portion of the event. (If you are going to see the latest science-fiction epic, see it in two or more sessions. This may seem extreme, but you are asking for trouble if you expect an STNR child to sit quietly through a four-hour event. The child won't enjoy the event any more than you will.)
- Refer to the list of general circumventions for public situations on pages 126–27.
- Be as pleasant and patient as possible.

Remember: we *are not* recommending unguided permissiveness, nor are we recommending that your STNR child be given postural freedom at the expense of the comfort of other people. We are recommending that you allow your child to be comfortable within the limits imposed by respect for other people's space and quiet. Ideally, the reflex can be matured through professional diagnosis, training, and monitoring at the Miriam Bender Achievement Center in Indianapolis, Indiana. If it is not possible to attend the Miriam Bender Achievement Center, the reflex can be matured through the exercise program described in Part Three of this book. Maturation of the STNR will eliminate the need for the modifications or circumventions. Until that time, these circumventions can make life easier for all concerned.

Now you are aware of the numerous difficulties that can be caused by an immature STNR. With this new information as a guide, it becomes your opportunity and your responsibility to analyze tasks that seem difficult for your children. Become a detective. Ask, "Why isn't my child succeeding quickly in a task that seems so simple?" Identifying the real problem is essential before anyone can possibly choose appropriate remediation.

Not all academic or behavioral problems are caused by an immature STNR. However, many of these most common problems are initially caused by or compounded by the STNR. Learned behavior traits or habits, such as avoidance tactics, defense mechanisms, and refusal or reluctance to do written work, may have become ingrained over the years. Removing the interfering effects of the STNR will not necessarily change these habits immediately. Occasionally, after the STNR is matured, academic remediation and behavioral management techniques are necessary to help the child more fully reach his or her potential. But if the basic difficulty is an immature STNR, all the academic remediation and behavioral techniques in the world will not get the job done until the reflex is matured.

You can help the child bridge the time between maturing the reflex and developing new habits by using some of the circumventions in Part Two. Gradually, the child will realize that it is no longer necessary to use the old avoidance tactics or to commit abnormal amounts of time to a task. Easier success will usually create better attitudes toward academic tasks and acceptable behaviors. The greatest motivator is success!

If your child is having problems in public situations, consider that the major problem may be an immature STNR.

Read on to discover how to mature the STNR.

General Circumventions for Public Situations

Throughout this chapter, we discuss numerous circumventions specific to various public situations. The more general circumventions presented below will allow STNR children to function more comfortably in public.

- Allow postural freedom to the extent that safety and the social situation will permit. Remember that an STNR child is more comfortable standing or lying down than sitting up straight, and that he or she needs to get up and change position to relieve the tension that the reflex causes. Do not require the child to sit unless it is absolutely necessary, which is actually rare. Think about it.

- Provide as much room for the child as possible. Since the STNR child needs to change position to relieve tension, choose a location where the child has room to move and can move without disturbing other people. It would be wise to choose a roomy van over a small car, aisle seats over seats in the middle of a row, and a restaurant table in an unobtrusive corner rather than one in the center of the room.

- Keep activities short or provide frequent breaks during longer activities. You are asking for trouble if you expect an STNR child to sit quietly through an event lasting an hour. The child won't enjoy the event any more than you will.

- Try to minimize waiting time. If a wait must be endured, allow the child to take a walk until the wait is over.
- Try not to worry about what other people think so long as your child is not being disruptive to the point of annoyance. If you feel comfortable doing so, try to explain how uncomfortable STNR children are, or give disapproving observers a copy of this book.
- Take quiet games, toys, or activities for your child to play with while waiting.
- Avoid or modify activities that are almost certain to cause trouble. Choose an informal restaurant over a formal one, a sing-along over a classical recital, a hands-on art workshop over a seated lecture until you have matured the STNR.
- Be as pleasant and patient as possible. We cannot stress this enough.

PART THREE

How to Solve the Real Problem

We know that the STNR exercises described in chapter 9 will solve the STNR problem if they are done properly. We know this because the clinical work done by Dr. Bender at Purdue University, and our own clinical programs at the University of Indianapolis and at the Miriam Bender Achievement Center (Indianapolis, Indiana) have demonstrated that these exercises will mature the immature STNR. "The good news is that movement activities that take children back through these missed stages and fundamental patterns can often correct flaws in their perceptual processes and enhance learning." (Gilbert 2001)

An STNR remains immature when a child does not crawl enough or does not crawl properly. The following exercises will provide sufficient and proper crawling to mature the reflex within eight months.*

The STNR exercises will significantly help anyone (child or adult) who:

* Note: We have extended the length of time for the STNR exercise program from a minimum of 6½ months in the first edition to a minimum of 8 months in this second edition. We have found that unless people have our professional input, they are more inconsistent in implementing the program; therefore, an extension of time should be of benefit.

- spent too much time in a playpen or walker
- wore leg braces or casts during the crawling stage
- walked early (before the age of one year)
- for whatever reason, did not crawl properly as an infant
- for whatever reason, did not crawl long enough (for at least six months) as an infant

The STNR exercises will also help anyone who displays one or more of the following behaviors as a result of an immature STNR:

- squirming
- sitting "inappropriately"
- getting up frequently
- losing attention quickly
- daydreaming frequently
- writing poorly or illegibly
- writing laboriously
- reversing letters or numbers
- moving awkwardly or clumsily
- avoiding athletics or developing athletic skills slowly

Not all of these behaviors have to be present to indicate the interfering effects of the immature STNR. One may be sufficient.

How do we solve the problem of an immature STNR? Again, we emphasize that these exercises will mature the STNR if they are done properly. Please follow the directions carefully, or make an appointment at our clinic.

If you can come to the Miriam Bender Achievement Center (see page 186 for contact information), it will be easier to properly implement these exercises through professional supervision. At our clinic our professional monitoring of each client's progress every six to eight weeks and making modifications specific to each individual's needs and rate of improvement will help to ensure the success of the program. In our many years of experience, there has *always* been *sig-*

nificant improvement in every case where the STNR exercise program has been implemented correctly and completed.

If you have not read the previous two parts of the book, please do so now. A thorough understanding of the STNR reflex and of the problems created by an immature STNR is essential as you work through the exercise program.

9. The STNR Exercises

This exercise program is designed to significantly increase the attention span, comfort, and efficiency of anyone who is hampered by an immature STNR. The program consists of specific crawling exercises and other developmental exercises that take about fifteen to twenty minutes a day, five days a week. The program should last for approximately eight months. Children need to be at least five years old to perform these exercises, but there is no upper age limit. Any adult or child over five years of age who has an immature STNR can benefit from these exercises.

"A reflex stimulation/inhibition program aims to give the brain a 'second chance' to experience the movements that should have been made in the early months of development. It thereby creates a bridge between the gaps and facilitates more efficient transmission and execution of messages passing between the brain and the body. Whereas many other methods of intervention work from the cortex *down* towards the brain stem, reflex stimulation and inhibition programs start from the spinal cord and brain stem and work *up* towards the cortex to access improved cortical control by providing more efficient pathways." (Goddard 2002, p. 124)

These exercises require the interaction of two people: the person with an immature STNR and another individual who provides physical resistance throughout the exercises (see "Use of Resistance in the

The STNR Test

At the Miriam Bender Achievement Center, we use the STNR test developed by Dr. Miriam L. Bender to help us determine if a child or adult is being affected by an immature STNR. In this reflex test, the child or adult performs crawling exercises as a trained clinician applies physical resistance. As the client performs the exercises, evaluations of body postures, body positions, rhythm, and coordination are rated by a second trained clinician, and a score ranging from 0 to 96 is assigned. The higher the score, the more interfering the STNR is considered to be. The reflex is deemed to be at an interfering level when the score is 40 to 41, or higher. When scores are borderline, information is gathered through interviews with the client and his or her parents and teachers to help determine if the STNR is at an interfering level, and if the STNR exercise program would be of benefit.

STNR Exercises" on page 143). The exercises can be done at any time and at any place that is twenty feet long and as wide as your body. Missing an occasional day of exercises will not significantly interfere with the program. However, if the occasional day of missed exercises accumulates to a week or more, the missed exercises should be made up by extending the exercise program. Add days at the end rather than "doubling up" in one day.

Getting Ready

To implement the STNR exercises, you will need the following:

- A straight stretch of floor twenty to twenty-five feet long. (You can crawl from one room into another, if need be, to create the necessary amount of space.) It should be wide enough for your body when you are in a crawling position. It should also be carpeted or padded if possible. Hallways are good areas. If there is no carpeting, a remnant carpet strip will work.

- Kneepads if the area is not carpeted or not sufficiently padded. *Do not crawl with unprotected knees* on linoleum, hardwood, indoor-outdoor carpeting, or any other non-padded surface. Soft, cushioned volleyball kneepads work exceptionally well. Kneepads for wrestling, skating, or carpentry will serve, or you can make kneepads from foam or potholders. Do not use hard kneepads.
- Two targets, one for each end of the crawling runway. They should be brightly colored and six to eight inches in size. For children who are really having trouble keeping their heads up, using a mirror or TV or another person waving a puppet as targets can be beneficial.
- Long, loose-fitting pants (not shorts and not tight jeans).
- Socks (but not shoes).

General Directions

Before beginning the STNR exercises, make a list of all the difficulties that the child is experiencing—in essence, why you feel the need to do these exercises. It is important to have a record of these problems to use as a baseline of behavior. *Do not* share this list with your child, for it could seem fault-finding and nit-picky. Put the list away where you can find it after you have completed the STNR exercise program.

When you have completed the STNR exercises (in approximately eight months) retrieve the list of the previous eight months' difficulties and compare it to your child's current behaviors. You will be amazed at how many of the problems either no longer exist or are significantly lessened. Please make this list.

Parents/crawling partners should keep the following guidelines in mind when conducting any of the STNR exercises:

- Do these exercises only with individuals five years of age or older.

- Listen to what the child tells you! You will be providing resistance during all of the exercises. If the child says that you are pushing or pulling too much (giving too much resistance), or that the resistance hurts, *you must let up!* Occasionally, parents do not provide enough resistance. How much is enough? The child is the only one who can really tell you how much is enough. Ask the child if the amount of resistance feels all right. This is not a contest of strength. The child should *work just a little harder* than if you were not giving resistance at all.

- Do the exercises when the child is rested or at least not seriously fatigued.

- Choose the time of day when the child functions best.

- Do the exercises five days a week for approximately eight months. The exercises take about fifteen to twenty minutes a day. (If you finish in less than ten minutes, you are crawling too fast.)

- Schedule the exercises. Although the child does not have to do them at the same time each day, you should establish a schedule for them. (If you plan to do them "when you get around to it," you will never get around to it.)

- Help your child make and mark a calendar to show that the exercises have been done five times per week. Stickers are great for this.

- At the end of each week, give the child an appropriate inexpensive reward. You might take a walk together, play a game, share a special nutritious treat, or give the child a small toy or an added allowance. Older children may enjoy putting money in a fund for a larger reward at the completion of the exercise program, but younger children need more frequent encouragement. "Eight months from now" is meaningless to young children.

- Keep the child focused on the task at hand during the exercise time. This should be a work session, but a pleasant one. If other children are distracting factors, they should not be in the room during exercise time. (Expect some sibling rivalry from your other children in reaction to the one-on-one attention you will be giving to the STNR child. Giving each of your other children a few minutes of their own one-on-one time will reassure them that you still love them, too, and will significantly reduce the sibling rivalry.)

- If you decide to have siblings be the crawling partners, be certain that you personally monitor the exercise sessions.
- Keep all verbal directions short, simple, and positive. Tell the child what he or she *should* do rather than what *not* to do. Avoid unnecessary chitchat during the actual exercises, at least during the first few months.
- If the child seems overly hesitant, nervous, or reluctant to try something so new and different as these exercises, demonstrate the exercises on another person first.
- At the beginning of the exercise program, the child's neck may hurt from holding the head up. A brief neck rub or massage should help. The sooner the child succeeds in raising the head and keeping it up, the sooner these aches will go away. If the child is still experiencing significant neck discomfort or trouble raising the head after the first six weeks, we recommend consulting a chiropractor or osteopath for appropriate physical adjustments to alleviate the pain and help with keeping the head up. Although chiropractic or osteopathic adjustments will not mature the reflex, they may facilitate the child's ability to implement the program.
- Some children may complain that their wrists hurt. This usually does not last very long. In the meantime, have them shake their hands back and forth a few times or rub their wrists for them.
- Be as pleasant and patient as possible. These exercises will be difficult for the individuals who need to do them. If they could do the exercises easily and perfectly from the beginning, they would not need to do them at all.

STNR 32-Week Exercise Program

WEEK	1	2	3	4	5	6	7	8	9	10	11	12	13	14	15	16	

STNR EXERCISES

Resisted Rocking
30 Cycles

Crawling I
6 round-trips

Modification for Crawling I 3 round-trips

Crawling II
3 round-trips

Week 9

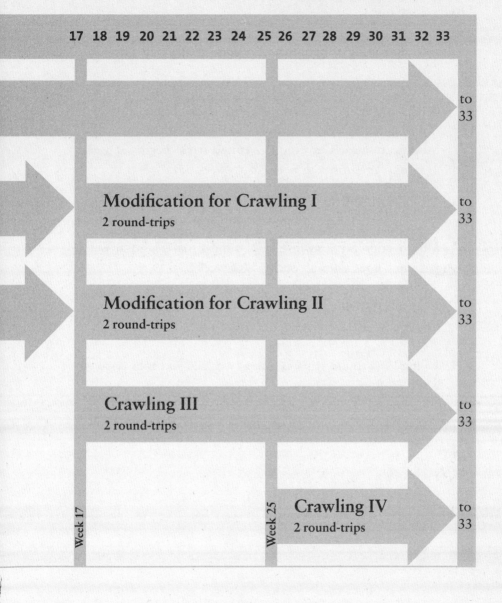

For those of you who prefer reading the directions, here are the time-lines written out:

Resisted rocking goes from week 1 *through* week 32 (to week 33).

Crawling I (6 round-trips) goes from week 1 *through* week 8.
   Modification for Crawling I (3 round-trips) begins at week 9 and goes *through* week 16.
   Modification for Crawling I (2 round-trips) begins at week 17 and goes *through* week 32 (to week 33).

Crawling II (3 round-trips) begins at week 9 and goes *through* week 16.
   Modification for Crawling II (2 round-trips) begins at week 17 and goes *through* week 32 (to week 33).

Crawling III (2 round-trips) begins at week 17, and goes *through* week 32 (to week 33).

Crawling IV (2 round-trips) begins at week 25 and goes *through* week 32 (to week 33).

The Exercises

The STNR exercise program* begins with two exercises, Resisted Rocking and Crawling I. These exercises are continued throughout the regimen, with modification, and others are added at eight week intervals. Please note that the exercises are presented below in the order in which they are introduced into the program. (See the chart on pages 138–139 for an overview of the program.) Every exercise begins with the box position, which is described directly below.

The Box Position

THE BEGINNING POSITION FOR ALL EXERCISES

All of the exercises begin from a position that we call the "box position."

- Have the child, or whoever needs these exercises, get on hands and knees in a crawling position.
- The arms should be straight down from the shoulders, *hands flat* on the floor and pointing directly ahead.
- The knees should be directly below the hips, with the *lower legs and feet extended flat* on the floor behind.
- The stomach should be off the floor.
- The head should be held up, with the face looking straight ahead, and the chin parallel to the floor. Holding the head up can be very uncomfortable in the beginning for STNR individuals, but it is *essential* that the head be up. (Do not make them throw their heads clear back in an unnatural extension of the neck.) Lifting the head to look straight forward should cause a slight sway or dip in the child's back. That is all right. However, arching (raising) the back interferes with keeping the head up. Lightly tap in the middle of the back and say, "Relax right here," or "Let

* A supplementary video or DVD that demonstrates the STNR exercises is available. See page 186 for contact information.

your stomach drop down a little." Do not do these exercises with the back arched (raised). (See figure 9.1 for the correct position; see figures 9.2 and 9.3 for incorrect positions.)

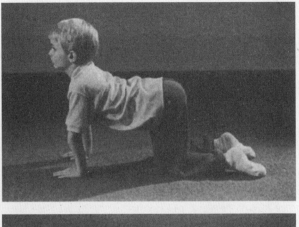

FIGURE 9.1.
Correct Box Position

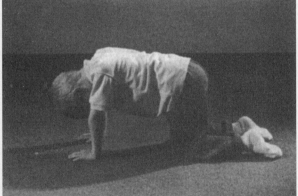

FIGURE 9.2.
Incorrect Box Position

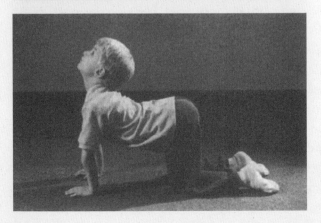

FIGURE 9.3.
Incorrect Box Position

Use of Resistance in the STNR Exercises

When Dr. Miriam Bender developed the exercises designed to mature the STNR, she included resistance (sometimes called stress) to maximize and hasten the results. Her research (Bender 1976) indicated that free or non-stressful crawling did not seem to be sufficient for the child to mature this reflex. The child apparently either did not receive enough proprioceptive feedback or did not benefit from the feedback sufficiently to allow a normal developmental progression. Proprioceptive feedback is the sensation from active muscles and joints that provides information about limb positions and movements of parts of the body. This feedback is monitored and utilized by an individual for production of more accurate responses. Dr. Bender emphasized the importance of adequate and consistent proprioceptive feedback to a child's motor development (Bender 1971). Intensifying the proprioceptive feedback should help with motor development.

Milner (1970) and Merton (1972) both reported that neurons fire faster in direct relationship to the amount of tension or force to be exerted by the associated muscle. Consequently, as neuronal efficiency increases through frequency of use, and as neurons fire faster as more force is applied to the associated muscles, resisted exercises should help to develop the appropriate neural pathways more quickly than nonresisted exercises would.

Neurological theory and functioning both indicate the importance of proprioceptive feedback to proper motor development. Neural efficiency seems related to the frequency of use of neural pathways, and stress of a force on a muscle creates more rapid firing of the associated neurons. Consequently, Dr. Bender found that the utilization of resistance enhanced the effectiveness of the crawling exercises.

Resisted Rocking

The Resisted Rocking Exercise begins the program to mature the immature STNR. This exercise is continued throughout the exercise program.

1. Sit on the floor with your back against a wall and your legs spread out.
2. Have the child get into the box position, backed up close in front of you, facing away from you and looking at a target at least six feet away. (Watching a TV during this exercise can help keep the head up.) (See figure 9.4.)

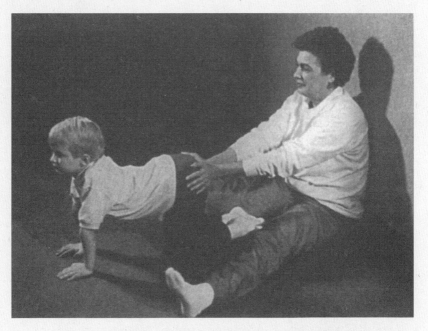

FIGURE 9.4. **Beginning Rocking Position**

3. Place your hands sideways on the broadest part of the child's bottom. (See figure 9.5.)

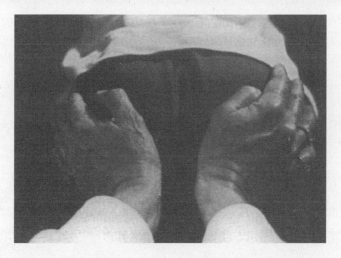

FIGURE 9.5. **Correct Hand Placement**

4. Make certain the child's head is up, the hands flat with fingers pointed straight forward, the feet flat with the toes pointed straight back. (See figure 9.6.)

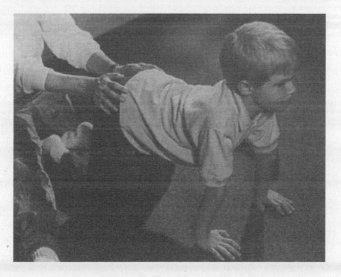

FIGURE 9.6. **Correct Box Position**

5. Say, "Rock back." (Do not just say, "Go.") Apply slight pressure (resistance) as the child rocks backward, sitting completely down on his flattened feet. (See figure 9.7.) Be sure to give this verbal direction *each time*. The child should not move until *after* you have *completed* the verbal direction. Make certain you are not pushing too hard. (Ask the child.)

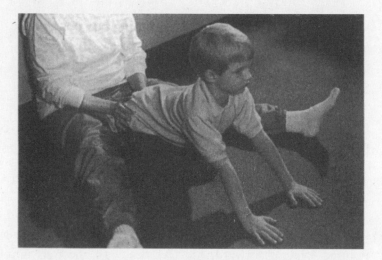

FIGURE 9.7. **Sitting Down on Feet**

6. The child's hands are to remain stationary (still) as the child sits back (all the way down) onto the heels. If this stretched-out position is too uncomfortable for the child, the head cannot stay up (figure 9.8). If this is the case, the child's hands should be pulled in slightly closer to the child's knees, thereby relieving the undue

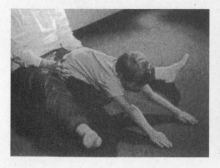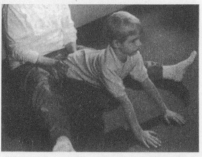

FIGURE 9.8. **Incorrect Position**   FIGURE 9.9. **Correct Position**

tension on the body and making it easier to maintain the correct head position (figure 9.9). Make certain that the child does not bring the hands too close to the knees. There must be enough space maintained between the hands and knees for an adequate rocking motion. Once this adjustment is made, the child's hands should remain stationary throughout this exercise.

7. Have the child hold this position for one full second.
8. Say, "Rock forward." (Do not just say, "Go.") You can remove your hands from the child's bottom during the forward motion, or leave your hands on but do *not* push the child forward. Be sure to give this verbal direction *each time*. The child should not move until *after* you have *completed* the verbal direction.
9. The child rocks forward, into the beginning box position (figure 9.10).

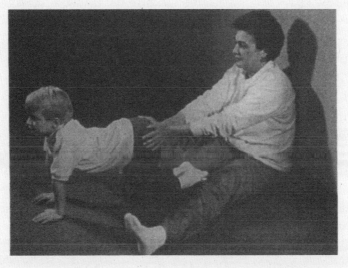

FIGURE 9.10. **Beginning Box Position**

10. Have the child hold this position for one full second.
11. Make certain the head is up and the hands and feet stay flat. You may need to have another person hold the child's hands flat, gently but firmly; or you can place a heavy book on the hands to help keep them flat. You may also need to sit lightly on the child's toes to help keep the feet flat, leaving enough space for the child to sit totally down on the flattened feet.

12. One cycle of rocking consists of rocking back onto the feet and then up into the box position.

Important Points

- *Make certain that the child's head stays up.* The upright head position is *essential* to each of the exercises. Rocking for eight months with the head down will not mature the reflex. Even though you are sitting behind the child, you can tell if the head is up by the position of the ears, or a cowlick, or a hair barrette, or some other clue. The STNR tends to pull the child's head down. Without sounding angry, you must keep reminding the child to keep the head up. Saying, "Lift your chin," will help most children to keep their heads up.
- *The child must hold each position for a full second.*
- *Give a verbal direction each time.* Even if the child says the repetition is not necessary, continue with the verbal direction.
- *Tell the child which direction to move* ("Rock forward" or "Rock backward") to help establish a better sense of direction. Do not just say, "Go."
- *The child must not move until after you have completed the verbal direction.*
- *Do not push too hard* (ask the child).
- *Be as pleasant and patient as possible.*

🕒 Repeat this exercise for thirty cycles (thirty times) in a row, five days a week for eight weeks, along with the next exercise, Crawling I. If thirty repetitions are too exhausting for the child, do two sessions of fifteen repetitions, or three sessions of ten repetitions. *You must begin at a stage where the child can be successful.*

Variations on Rocking

For the child who does not seem able to move against even the slightest bit of physical pressure, try letting the child do "free" rocking (with no physical pressure) for several weeks to practice the rocking motion. Add slight physical pressure to the Rocking Exercise when the child can successfully push against it.

For the child who is uncomfortable being touched (tactile defensiveness), try placing a gardener's kneeling pad, or a small pillow, or a piece of foam rubber between the child's bottom and your hands.

Crawling I (Shoulder Resistance)

We are going to describe two ways to do this exercise. Choose either method, whichever is more comfortable for you and your child.

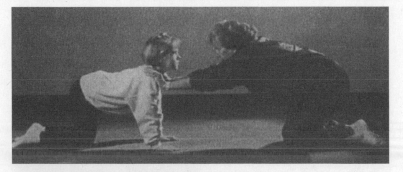

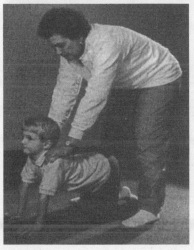

(▲) METHOD A, for children large enough to balance a portion of their parent's weight.

(◄) METHOD B, for smaller children or for children with large parents.

Like Resisted Rocking, this exercise begins at the start of the program.

METHOD A

We recommend Method A for children who are large enough to balance a portion of their parent's weight.

1. Have the child get into the Box Position at one end of the runway, facing the target at the other end of the runway. (Make certain that the child's head is up, and feet and hands are flat, fingers pointing straight ahead.)
2. Facing the child, kneel down and put your hands on the child's shoulders. Straighten your arms and lock your elbows. Make certain your palms are flat (thumbs alongside your fingers, not pushing on the collarbone) and push *straight into* the child's shoulders, not down on the shoulders (see figure 9.11).

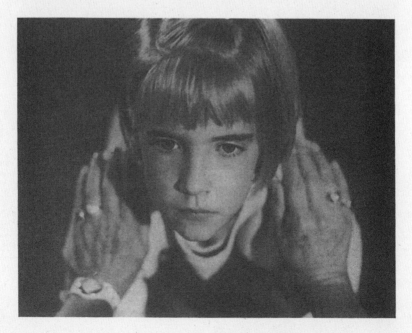

FIGURE 9.11. **Correct Hand Position—
Pushing Into the Shoulders**

3. Stretch out so that your nose is at the same height as the child's nose (see figure 9.12). (Your nose is the child's target for this exercise.) *Keep your nose down at the child's level,* or the child is likely to rise up on thumbs and fingers in order to watch your nose (see figure 9.13).

4. Say, "Crawl forward." Give slight resistance into the child's shoulders. Crawl backward as the child moves forward, maintaining the slight resistance into the child's shoulders. (The child

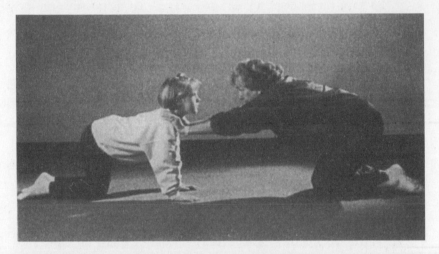

FIGURE 9.12. **Correct Position**

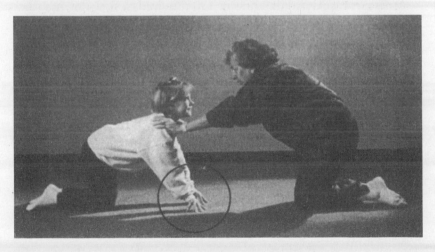

FIGURE 9.13. **Incorrect Position**

should crawl smoothly and without extreme effort. If that is not happening, you are pushing too hard. Let up on the resistance! Pay attention to what the child "tells" you through grunts, groans, amount of effort exerted, wobbliness, and other clues. Ask the child if the amount of resistance feels all right. You will soon develop a sense of the right amount of resistance to apply.) This is not a contest of strength, but you must apply some slight resistance.

5.   Keep *your* knees, legs, ankles, and feet as flat as possible on the floor as you crawl backward. Otherwise, your balance will be very shaky as you crawl backward on just your kneecaps, making you lean on the child for your balance. (See figures 9.14 and 9.15.)

Important Points

- Make *certain* that the child's head stays up. Do not nag, but you may say, "Lift your chin" or "Watch my nose" two or three times a trip if necessary.
- *Once* each trip you may say, "Flatten your hands" or "Point with your fingers straight ahead." (Too many directions will drive the child crazy.)
- Each trip up and down the runway should be relatively slow and smooth. The child should not be allowed to "explode" into movement or race down the runway. Tell the child to slow down, rather than add more resistance to reduce the speed. A single trip down the twenty-foot runway should take fifteen to twenty seconds. From one end of the runway and back again is one round-trip.
- These exercises should not cause pain. Ask the child. If the child says that something is hurting, let up on the resistance or readjust your hand position on the child's body.
- Be as pleasant and patient as possible.

☉ Do six round-trips, five days a week for eight weeks along with the Rocking Exercise. (An option is to do three round-trips of Crawling I, then fifteen rockers, then three round-trips of Crawling I and then fifteen rockers.)

If the child cannot do a total of six round-trips of Crawling I

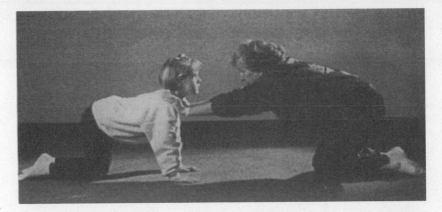

FIGURE 9.14. **Correct Position**

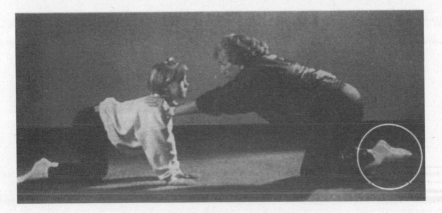

FIGURE 9.15. **Incorrect Position**

correctly and fairly smoothly then try for a total of three round-trips. If even that amount seems too difficult, do not do Crawling I now. Do only the Rocking Exercise for eight weeks. Then again try adding Crawling I for eight weeks and continue with the Rocking Exercise.

Do not worry if the child cannot do this first crawling exercise at the beginning of the exercise program. Doing the Rocking Exercise alone, successfully, for eight weeks should prepare the child for Crawling I, even if on a reduced basis. This program *will work,* but *you must begin at a stage where the child can be successful.*

Variations on Crawling I (Method A)

For the child who can do the Rocking Exercise but who cannot crawl against the slightest bit of physical pressure, try letting the child do "free" crawling (with no physical pressure) for several weeks to practice the crawling movements. Continue with the Rocking Exercise. Add slight physical pressure to Crawling I when the child can successfully crawl against the pressure.

METHOD B

We usually recommend Method B for smaller children or for children with large parents.

1. Have the child get into the Box Position at one end of the runway, facing the target at the other end of the runway. (Make certain that the child's head is up, and feet and hands are flat, fingers pointing straight ahead.)

2. Stand over the child's back (straddle the child) facing the same direction as the child. Lean over slightly and stretch your arms down, placing your hands on the front of the child's shoulders. You should be able to see the end of the child's nose when the child's head is sufficiently up if your body is adequately forward. Your body should be farther forward over the child's body than is indicated in figure 9.16. Your feet should be beside the child's shoulders. If the child's nose goes out of sight, you will know the head has dropped too low.

3. Say, "Crawl forward." Give *slight* resistance, pulling backward into the child's shoulders, walking forward as the child crawls forward. *Do not* dig into the child's shoulders. *Do not* pull upward on the child's shoulders. (See figure 9.17.)

4. If the child is very small, or if you have large, heavy hands, use only one or two fingers on each shoulder for resistance. Ask the child if the amount of resistance feels all right.

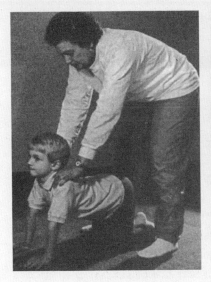

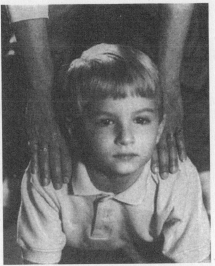

FIGURE 9.16. **Side View**   FIGURE 9.17. **Front View**

Important Points

- Make *certain* that the child's head stays up. Do not nag, but you may say, "Lift your chin" or "Watch the target," two or three times a trip if necessary.

- *Once* each trip you may say, "Flatten your hands" or "Point with your fingers straight ahead." (Too many directions will drive the child crazy.)

- Each trip up and down the runway should be relatively slow and smooth. The child should not be allowed to "explode" into movement or race down the runway. Tell the child to slow down, rather than add more resistance to reduce the speed. A single trip down the twenty-foot runway should take fifteen to twenty seconds. From one end of the runway and back again is one round-trip.

- These exercises should not cause pain. Ask the child. If the child says that something is hurting, let up on the resistance or readjust your hand position on the child's body.

- Be as pleasant and patient as possible.

⏱ Do six round-trips, five days a week for eight weeks along with the Rocking Exercise. (An option is to do three round-trips of Crawling I, then fifteen rockers, then three round-trips of Crawling I and then fifteen rockers.)

If the child cannot do a total of six round-trips of Crawling I correctly and fairly smoothly, then try for a total of three round-trips. If even that amount seems too difficult, do not do Crawling I now. Do only the Rocking Exercise for eight weeks. Then again try adding Crawling I for eight weeks and continue with the Rocking Exercise.

Do not worry if the child cannot do this first crawling exercise at the beginning of the exercise program. Doing the Rocking Exercise alone, successfully, for eight weeks should prepare the child for Crawling I, even if on a reduced basis. This program *will work*, but *you must begin at a stage where the child can be successful.*

Variations on Crawling I (Method B)

For the child who can do the Rocking Exercise but who cannot crawl against the slightest bit of physical pressure, try letting the child do "free" crawling (with no physical pressure) for several weeks to practice the crawling movements. Continue with the Rocking Exercise. Add slight physical pressure to Crawling I when the child can successfully crawl against the pressure.

For the child who is uncomfortable being touched (tactile defensiveness) or for the parent who cannot comfortably lean over (figure 9.16), resistance can be applied in other ways. Loop a separate towel under each of the child's arms and over each shoulder, bringing the extended towels together behind the child in somewhat of a harness fashion. The parent can then walk behind the child pulling gently backward, not upward, on the towels, giving slight resistance to the child's shoulders. Do not restrict the child's arm movements. Another possibility is to put an oversized sweatshirt on the child. The parent stands behind the child and pulls backward, not

upward, on the bottom half of the sweatshirt, giving slight resistance as the child crawls forward. (Notice we say *slight* resistance.
The child needs to be able to breathe to do this exercise.)

Crawling II (Ankle Pull)

After eight weeks of Rocking and Crawling I, add the Crawling II
(Ankle Pull) exercise for eight weeks and Modification for Crawling I
(see page 163).

1. Have the child get into the Box Position at one end of the runway,
    facing the target at the other end of the runway. (Make certain
    that the child's head is up, feet and hands are flat, fingers point-
    ing straight ahead.)
2. Get into the Box Position directly behind the child (see figure 9.18).

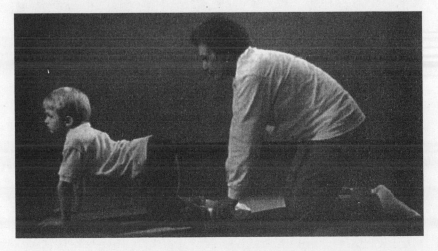

FIGURE 9.18. **Crawling II Beginning Position**

3. Select the child's leg that you want to be moved first; pat or shake
    that leg and say, "Move this leg first when I say to pull." (If the

child seems to prefer starting with a particular leg, then pat that leg and begin with it.)

4. Option 1: Grasp the child's ankle bones; put your middle finger on the outside ankle bone and your thumb on the inside ankle bone, cupping the child's heel in the curvature of your palm. Turn your wrists slightly inward, toward each other (see figure 9.19).

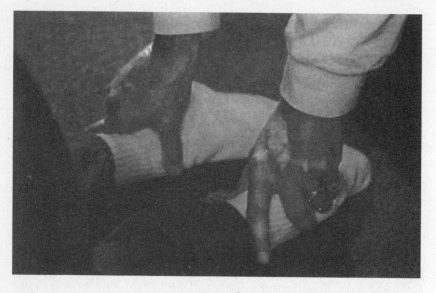

FIGURE 9.19. **Option 1**

Option 2: Spread your thumb from your fingers and cup the child's heel in the "V" between your thumb and fingers. Hold firmly but do not squeeze the heel or any other part of the foot (see figure 9.20).

Option 3: If Options 1 and 2 cause physical discomfort for the child, you may hold on to the leg bones or the feet, as long as you do not squeeze them or lift them off the floor.

5. *You* must keep the child's feet as flat as possible on the floor. Turning the child's toes somewhat inward toward each other and the ankles outward (so that the child's position is "pigeon-toed") will help to keep the child's feet as flat as possible. Keeping the feet flat against the floor does not mean adding extra resistance (see figure 9.21).

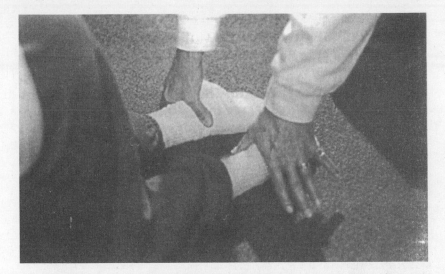

FIGURE 9.20. **Option 2**

6. Say, "Pull." As you give this verbal direction, tug the ankle bones (Option 1) or heels (Option 2) of the leg you have indicated the child is to begin with. This should be a "rebound tug," one quick pull back and forth. The verbal cue and the rebound tug should be *given simultaneously each time* the child is to move a leg.

7. The child should move just *one hand* with each forward leg motion. Do *not* tell the child which hand to move.

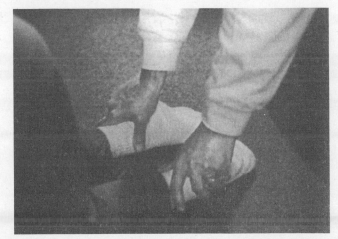

FIGURE 9.21. **Keeping the Feet Flat**

8. Pull slightly backward on the ankle, giving some resistance, as the child slides forward the leg you indicated. The child should have to work just a little harder than if you were not giving any resistance at all. (You may have to lean slightly backward to apply enough resistance for larger children.) Ask the child if the amount of resistance feels all right.

9. Remember: Say, "Pull," and simultaneously give the rebound tug alternately to each leg every time the child is to take a crawling step.

10. You should take a crawling step forward each time the child moves forward. When the child moves the left leg, you move your left leg, and so on (see figure 9.22). (Be careful not to crawl up onto the child's toes.)

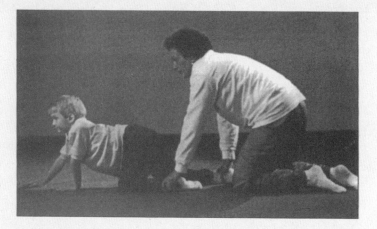

FIGURE 9.22. **Correct Crawling II Position**

11. Stop and pause for one full second after each forward step. *You* must set the pace and rhythm of the crawling. Do *not* let the child set the speed, because it would probably be too fast or too slow. *Make* the child wait for your simultaneous verbal and rebound tug signals each time. The child should not move until *after* you have *completed* your signal.

Important Points

• *Make certain that the child's head stays up.* By looking along the child's back and monitoring the tops of the child's ears or the position of a cowlick or a hair barrette, you should be able to determine whether the child's head is up.

- Once each trip you may say, "Flatten your hands" or "Point with your fingers straight ahead." (Too many directions will be too frustrating for the child.)
- The ideal step length consists of the child's sliding the ankle of the moving leg up to the knee of the other leg. If the step length is too short, wiggle the child's foot and say, "Take a longer step." If the child takes too long a step, pull the leg back until the ankle is beside the other knee and say, "Take a shorter step." Ankle to knee is about right for everybody. (See figures 9.23, 9.24, and 9.25.)
- Encourage the child to *slide* the knees and legs rather than picking them up with each crawling step. It is *your* job to keep the child's feet flat on the floor.
- Work for smoothness in sliding the legs and an even step length (ankle to knee). These movements should not be explosive.
- You must wait a full second after each sliding step before giving the next signal to move.
- *Simultaneously* give a rebound tug and say, "Pull," *before each step.* Even if the child says the repetition is not necessary, continue with the simultaneous tug and verbal cue.
- The child must not move until *after you have completed* the simultaneous tug and verbal cue.
- Do not pull too hard (ask the child).
- Be as pleasant and patient as possible.

☉ Do three round-trips of this exercise on the twenty-foot runway. Decrease the Crawling I Exercise to three round-trips. (This way you are maintaining six round-trips of crawling. This is no addition of work for the child, just more variety.) Maintain the Rocking Exercise. Do Rocking, Modification for Crawling I (see page 163, and Crawling II, five times a week for eight weeks. (Implement the Modification for Crawling I from now on.)

If the child cannot do this new Crawling II exercise correctly and fairly smoothly without a great deal of frustration (remember that it

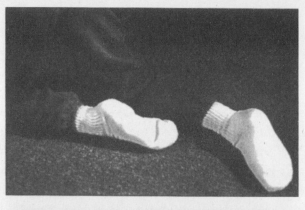

FIGURE 9.23.
Correct
Step Length

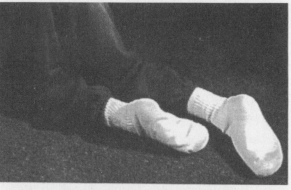

FIGURE 9.24.
Incorrect—Too
Short a Step

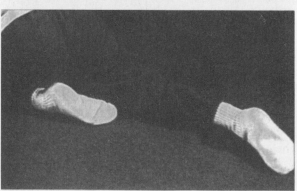

FIGURE 9.25.
Incorrect—Too
Long a Step

is new, so it will not be as easy to do), continue with the Rocking and
Modified Crawling I for another four weeks. Then again try adding
Crawling II for eight weeks while continuing Rocking and Modified
Crawling I.

Variations on Crawling II

For parents/crawling partners who cannot be on their knees, stand behind the child and bend over to hold on to the child's ankles. Make sure that you keep the child's feet flat on the floor. (You are more likely to pull the child's feet up off the floor when you are standing.) Continue with directions 3 through 11 and "Important Points."

MODIFICATION FOR CRAWLING I

After eight weeks of Rocking and Crawling I, the child should be able to hold his or her head up fairly well, and we can begin to pay more attention to the hand position. From now on, as the child crawls, with each forward movement of an arm, have the child bend the elbow of that arm so that the back of her hand gently hits the bottom of the parent's arm (Method A) or the child's corresponding shoulder (Method B). The child should lift the elbow, thrusting it up and out in front, toward the target. Do not let the elbow point down, or back, or out to the side like a chicken wing. (See figure 9.26 for the correction position; see figures 9.27 and 9.28 for incorrect positions.)

Then, as the child crawls forward, have the child *throw* the hand down (firmly, but not hard) and slap the floor. Bending the elbow and slapping the floor should help to flatten the hand and point the fingers straight ahead. Slapping the hand on the floor without first bending the elbow can jam the elbow and hurt like crazy. (If bending the elbows and slapping the hands cause the child's head to drop, delay this modification for eight weeks and just concentrate on keeping the child's head up and sliding the legs.) When the child can successfully lift the elbows and slap the hands down, add this modification and continue this modified form of the exercise for the remainder of the program.

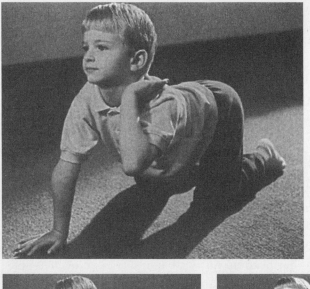

FIGURE 9.26.
Correct
Position

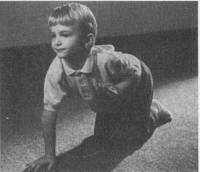

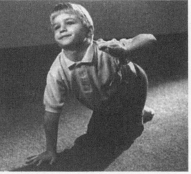

FIGURE 9.27. Incorrect Position   FIGURE 9.28. Incorrect Position

Crawling III (Heel Push)

After sixteen weeks of the previous exercises (eight weeks of Rocking and Crawling I, followed by eight weeks of Rocking, Modified Crawling I, and Crawling II), continue Rocking and Modified Crawling I and add the Crawling III (Heel Push) exercise for eight weeks and Modification for Crawling II (see page 169).

1.   Have the child get into the Box Position at one end of the runway, facing the target at *that* end of the runway. The child is going to

crawl backward. (Make certain that the child's head is up, feet and hands are flat, fingers pointing straight ahead.)

2. Get into the Box Position directly behind the child (see figure 9.29).

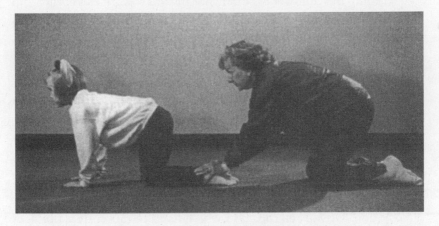

FIGURE 9.29. **Crawling III Beginning Position**

3. Place the heels of your *hands* against the heels of the child's *feet*. Back away enough so that you can straighten your arms and lock your elbows (see figure 9.30).

4. Select the leg that you want the child to move first, pat or shake that leg, and say, "Move this leg first when I say to push." (If the

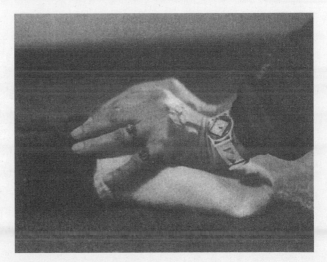

FIGURE 9.30.
**Correct Hand
Position**

child seems to prefer starting with a particular leg, then pat and
begin with that leg.)

5. *You* must keep the child's feet as flat as possible on the floor.
   Turning the child's toes somewhat inward toward each other and
   the ankles outward (so that the child's position is "pigeon-toed")
   will help to keep the child's feet as flat as possible. Keeping the
   feet flat against the floor does not mean adding extra resistance.

6. Say, "Push." As you give this verbal direction, simultaneously
   push firmly straight into the heel (not the arch) of the foot you
   have indicated the child is to begin with. This should be a "rebound push," (one quick push, then a relaxation). The verbal
   cue and the rebound push should be *given simultaneously each
   time* the child is to move a leg.

7. The child should move *just one hand* with each backward leg
   motion. Do *not* tell the child which hand to move. (It is not necessary for the child to bend the elbows and slap the hands when
   crawling backward. Let the child decide.)

8. Push forward into the child's heel, giving *slight* resistance, as the
   child slides backward the leg you indicated. The child should
   have to work just a little harder than if you were not giving any
   resistance at all. Caution: The child can *never* take as much resistance when going backward as when going forward. Remember, this is not a contest of strength. Ask the child if the amount
   of resistance feels all right.

9. Remember: Say, "Push," and simultaneously give the rebound
   push alternately to each leg every time the child is to take a
   crawling step.

10. You should take a crawling step backward each time the child
    moves backward. When the child moves the left leg, you move
    your left leg, and so on (see figure 9.31).

11. Stop and pause for one full second after each backward step. *You*
    must set the pace and rhythm of the crawling. Do *not* let the
    child set the speed, because it would probably be too fast or too
    slow. *Make* the child wait for your simultaneous verbal signal
    and rebound push each time. The child should not move until
    after you have *completed* your signal.

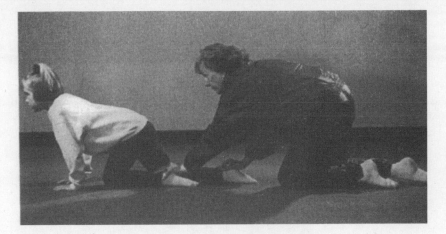

FIGURE 9.31. **Correct Step Length**

Important Points

- *Make certain that the child's head stays up.* By looking along the child's back and monitoring the tops of the child's ears or the position of a cowlick or a hair barrette, you should be able to determine whether the child's head is up.

- The ideal step length consists of the child's sliding the knee of the moving leg back to the ankle of the other leg. If the step length is too short, wiggle the child's foot and say, "Take a longer step." If the child takes too long a step, push the leg back until the knee is beside the other ankle and say, "Take a shorter step." Knee to ankle is about right for everybody (see figures 9.32 and 9.33).

- Encourage the child to slide the knees and legs rather than picking them up with each crawling step. It is *your* job to keep the child's feet flat on the floor.

- Work for smoothness in sliding the legs and an even step length (knee to ankle). These movements should not be explosive.

- You must wait a full second after each sliding step before giving the next signal to move.

- *Simultaneously* give a rebound push and say, "Push," *before each step.* Even if the child says the repetition is not necessary, continue with the simultaneous push and verbal cue.

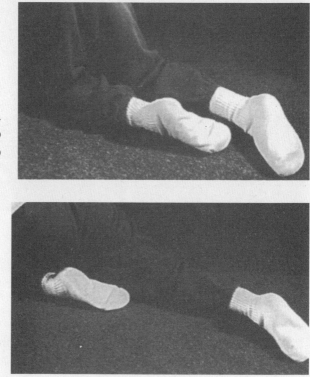

FIGURE 9.32.
Incorrect—Too
Short a Step

FIGURE 9.33.
Incorrect—
Too Long
a Step

- The child must not move until *after you have completed* the simultaneous push and verbal cue.
- Do not let the child drag both hands back while moving one leg. The child should move just one hand with each backward leg motion.
- Do not push too hard (ask the child).
- Be as pleasant and patient as possible.

☉ Do two round-trips of this exercise on the twenty-foot runway. Decrease the Modified Crawling I and Crawling II Exercises to two round-trips each. (This way you are maintaining six round-trips of crawling. This is no addition of work for the child, just more variety.) Maintain the Rocking Exercise. Do Rocking, Modified Crawling I, Modified Crawling II, and Crawling III, five times a week for eight weeks. (Implement the Modification for Crawling II from now on.)

If the child cannot do this new Crawling III exercise correctly and fairly smoothly, without a great deal of frustration (remember that it is new, so it will not be as easy to do), continue with the Rocking, Modified Crawling I and Modified Crawling II for another four weeks. Then again try adding Crawling III for eight weeks while continuing Rocking, Modified Crawling I, and Modified Crawling II.

Variations on Crawling III

For parents/crawling partners who cannot be on their knees, stand behind the child and bend over to push into the child's heels. Some crawling partners prefer to face the same direction as the child, walking backward as the child crawls backward. Some crawling partners prefer to face the opposite direction from the child, walking forward as the child crawls backward. Place your hands or fingertips against the child's heels to provide slight resistance. Continue with directions 4 through 11 and "Important Points."

MODIFICATION FOR CRAWLING II

Add the bending of elbows and slapping of hands on the floor to Crawling II now, in addition to Crawling I. From now on, as the child crawls, with each forward movement of an arm, have the child bend the elbow of that arm so that the back of that hand gently touches the corresponding shoulder. The child should lift the elbow, thrusting it up and out in front, toward the target. Do not let the elbow point down, or back, or out to the side like a chicken wing. (See figure 9.34 for the correct position; see figures 9.35 and 9.36 for incorrect positions.)

Then, as the child crawls forward, have the child throw the hand down (firmly, but not hard) and slap the floor. Bending the elbow and slapping the floor should help to flatten the hand and point the fingers straight ahead. Slapping the hand on the floor without first bending the elbow can jam the elbow and hurt like crazy. (If bending the elbows and slapping the hands cause the child's head to drop,

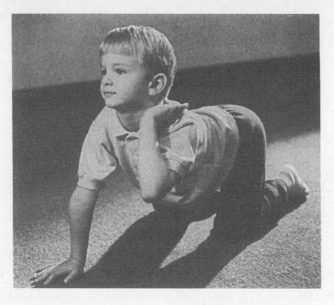

FIGURE 9.34. **Correct Position**

delay this modification for eight weeks and just concentrate on keeping the child's head up.) When the child can successfully lift the elbows and slap the hands down, add this modification and continue this modified form of the exercise for the remainder of the program. At this point in the exercise program, most children have developed a crawling pattern of moving an arm with the opposite leg (reciprocal) when crawling forward. However, if the child is still moving the arm

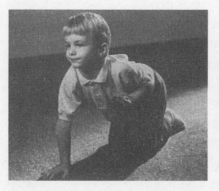
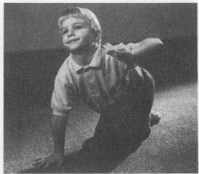

FIGURE 9.35. **Incorrect Position**   FIGURE 9.36. **Incorrect Position**

and leg on the same side (ipsilateral), you can try one of these approaches to ease the child into a reciprocal pattern:

1. tap the left hand and the right leg (or vice versa) at the beginning of the exercise;
2. position the child with the left hand and the right knee slightly forward (or vice versa) before beginning the exercise;
3. have the child lift the left elbow, thrusting it up and out in front, while waiting for the inital verbal cue, "Pull," and tug on the right leg (or vice versa).

Crawling in a reciprocal pattern is not a necessity. If s/he has developed a good rhythm, with a good step length, crawling in an ipsilateral pattern is acceptable.

These modifications are for *forward* crawling only. DO NOT impose a reciprocal pattern on backward crawling.

Crawling IV (Bottom Push)

After twenty-four weeks of the previous exercises (eight weeks of Rocking and Crawling I; followed by eight weeks of Rocking, Modified Crawling I, and Crawling II; followed by eight weeks of Rocking, Modified Crawling I, Modified Crawling II, and Crawling III), add the Crawling IV (Bottom Push) exercise for eight weeks.

1. Have the child get into the Box Position at one end of the runway, facing the target at that end of the runway. The child is going to crawl backward. (Make certain that the child's head is up, feet and hands are flat, fingers pointing straight ahead. At this point, some parents have found it beneficial to put some type of beanbag on the child's head to help keep the head up and steady.)
2. Get into the Box Position directly behind the child (see figure 9.37).
3. For a smaller child, place one of your hands in the middle of the child's bottom, using your other hand on the floor for balance (see figure 9.38). For a larger child, place both of your hands approx-

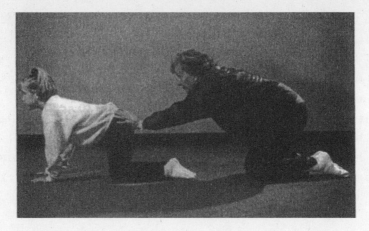

FIGURE 9.37. **Crawling IV Beginning Position**

imately three inches apart on the middle of the child's bottom. Back away enough so that you can straighten your arm or arms, providing slight resistance to the child's bottom (see figure 9.39).

4. Say, "Crawl backward." This verbal cue is to be given just once at the beginning of this exercise. The child is to crawl continuously, at a moderate pace, without stopping, and with no additional verbal cue.

5. Give slight resistance into the child's bottom. As the child crawls backward, you crawl backward, maintaining slight resistance on the child's bottom. When the child moves the left leg, you move

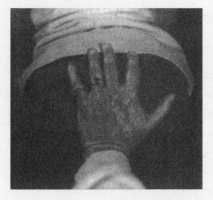

FIGURE 9.38. **One Hand for Smaller Child**

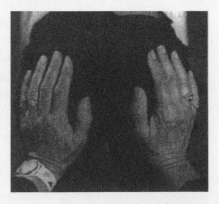

FIGURE 9.39. **Two Hands for Larger Child**

your left leg, and so on. Ask the child if the amount of resistance feels all right.

6. The child should move *just one hand* with each backward leg motion. Do not tell the child which hand to move. (It is not necessary for the child to bend the elbows and slap the hands when crawling backward. Let the child decide.)

7. In this exercise, it is the *child's* responsibility to keep the feet flat on the floor. It is *your* responsibility to monitor the child's feet. If the child's feet will not stay down, you are pushing too hard on the child's bottom, or going too fast, or the child is not yet ready for this exercise. If you let up on the resistance and slow down and still have to remind the child to keep the feet down more than once a trip after the first few days, discontinue this exercise. The child is not ready for it. Maintain the previous exercises for four more weeks and then try adding this exercise again.

Important Points

- *Make certain that the child's head stays up.* By looking along the child's back and monitoring the tops of the child's ears or the position of a cowlick or a hair barrette you should be able to determine whether the child's head is up.
- Encourage the ideal step length: from the knee of one leg to the ankle of the other leg.
- Encourage the child to slide the knees and legs rather than picking them up with each crawling step.
- Work for smoothness in sliding the legs and an even step length (knee to ankle). These movements should not be explosive and should be at a moderate pace.
- Do not let the child drag both hands back while moving one leg. The child should move *just one hand* with each backward leg motion.
- Make certain that the child's feet stay flat on the floor. If the child seems unable to keep the feet flat on the floor, refer back to Direction #7.
- Do not push too hard (ask the child).
- Be as pleasant and patient as possible.

🕐 Do two round-trips of this exercise on the twenty-foot runway. Maintain the Rocking, two round-trips each of Modified Crawling I, Modified Crawling II, and Crawling III, and add two round-trips of Crawling IV, five times a week for *eight* weeks.

If the child cannot do this new Crawling IV exercise correctly and fairly smoothly, without a great deal of frustration (remember that it is new, so it will not be as easy to do), continue with the Rocking, Modified Crawling I, Modified Crawling II, and Crawling III for another four weeks. Then again try adding Crawling IV for eight weeks while continuing Rocking, Modified Crawling I, Modified Crawling II, and Crawling III.

Variations on Crawling IV

For parents/crawling partners who cannot be on their knees, straddle the child or stand behind the child and bend over to push slightly on the child's bottom. Some crawling partners prefer to face the same direction as the child, walking backward as the child crawls backward. Some crawling partners prefer to face the opposite direction from the child, walking forward as the child crawls backward. Continue with directions 4 through 7 and "Important Points."

How to Know When the Reflex Is Matured

Please do not discontinue the STNR exercises halfway through just because the child shows improvement. If you are pleased with the improvements from doing half of the STNR exercises, you will be thrilled with the results gained from completing the entire program. It is important to complete the STNR program, including the gross and fine motor activities, to be sure the reflex is matured and integrated.

After you have done the STNR exercises for the amount of time recommended (approximately eight months), you should test the child to make certain that the reflex is mature before you stop the exercises. (Remember, the object of the STNR exercises is to mature the reflex, not just to make your child a good crawler.) When the reflex is mature, the child should be able to perform these exercises smoothly, with an even step length, with his or her head held up, feet flat on the floor, hands flat with fingers pointed straight ahead, while concentrating on something other than crawling.

Testing for Maturity of the STNR

Perform the Crawling IV exercise (Bottom Push) and ask the child to spell a word from an appropriate spelling list from the child's grade. *The reflex is not yet mature if*

- the child cannot crawl and spell simultaneously; instead, the child stops crawling, then spells, then start crawling again, *or*
- the child's head goes down while the child is spelling, *or*
- the child crawls and spells in cadence (one letter for each crawling step), *or*
- the child's general crawling performance deteriorates during the spelling.

If any one of these performances occurs, the reflex is *not mature*.

We are concerned with the crawling performance, not the spelling accuracy. (If the child misspells a word, wait until the exercise is finished before correcting the spelling.) Repeat this test two or three times for sufficient observation. Since you will be doing the exercise with the child, we recommend that you have someone else help with the observation of the child's performance.

Make sure that you provide your usual amount of resistance (no more and no less) during the test. Too much resistance can artificially cause deterioration of the crawling performance. Too little resistance does not provide adequate physical challenge for the crawling.

After eight months of the child's having done the exercises, if the reflex is not mature, continue two round-trips each of Crawling III (heel push) and Crawling IV (bottom push) for four more weeks, then retest. If the reflex is still not mature, continue Crawling III and IV for another four weeks.

The STNR is mature when the child can perform the Crawling IV exercise:

- smoothly,
- with an even step length,
- head up,
- feet flat on the floor,
- hands flat with fingers pointing straight ahead, *and*
- can spell words appropriate to the child's grade level out of cadence with the crawling, not with each letter "locked in" with each crawling step.

Once you are certain that the STNR is mature, a number of exercises can be used to further develop your child's coordination. Read on to learn about these simple exercises.

10. Exercises to Follow the Reflex Program

After the reflex program is completed, we recommend that you use the following exercises to further develop the child's gross motor and fine motor coordination. As P. Dennison and G. Dennison (1986) say in *Brain Gym,* "Whole brain learning through movement repatterning . . . enable(s) students to access those parts of the brain previously unavailable to them. The changes in learning and behavior are often immediate and profound as children discover how to receive information and express themselves simultaneously."

If the child is actively involved in a good physical education/athletic program, you may skip the following gross motor exercises and go directly to the fine motor exercises. (If you pass GO, collect $200.)

Gross Motor Exercises

Do these exercises for approximately ten minutes a day, five days a week, for six weeks. The exercises can be divided into two sessions if doing all of them at once is too strenuous for the child. It is generally better to do the exercises at regularly scheduled times. Monitor your child as she or he does these activities, looking for smoothness and ease. When both sides of the body are involved in the exercise, work on having your child use both sides equally. One side should not do most of the work. If your child tires easily at first, do only part of each exercise, but work toward the stated goals.

Toe Touch

Have the child touch the toes of both feet. The knees may be slightly bent. The hands should lower evenly. Work for a goal of ten, for children eight years old or younger; to fifteen, for older children.

Foot Touch

Have the child touch one foot with the opposite hand, then alternate hands and feet. The knees may be slightly bent. Work for a goal of ten, for children eight years old or younger; to fifteen, for older children.

Arm Twirls

Have the child make three large circles with both arms, keeping the elbows straight. The child should make circles in front, then at the sides, then over the head. Do four sets of these exercises. (Do two sets with circles going in one direction, then two with the circles going in the opposite direction.)

Side Bends

Have the child stand with feet apart. The child is to slide the right hand down the right leg as far as possible. Repeat with the left hand down the left leg. Alternate sides for a goal of ten bends on each side.

Side Twist

Have the child stand with feet apart and the arms straight out from the shoulders. Twisting from the waist, the child is to swing one arm out in front while the other swings toward the back, then reverse. Watch the child to see that the arms are kept at equal heights. (The front arm will go farther than the back arm.) Do ten sets of swings.

Kicking

Have the child, while standing, kick the right foot up to touch the left hand, then bring the left foot up to touch the right hand. Work for a goal of ten repetitions for each foot.

Balancing

Have the child balance on one foot for twenty seconds, then balance on the other foot for twenty seconds. (For children up to eight years of age, limit the balancing to ten seconds.) Repeat four times.

Fine Motor Exercises

After the completion of the crawling exercises and six weeks of gross motor exercises, move "up the motor ladder" to these fine motor exercises, which will help establish the proper motions for handwriting. The criteria are, as always, success and ease of production. When the child can successfully and relatively easily make the words or "letters," move to the next part of the program. You must be with the child throughout these exercises to make certain that they are done correctly.

- Use a large chalkboard. It should be three to four feet wide and about two feet high. You can make one from plywood or plasterboard, painting it with chalkboard paint, which is available at hardware stores.
- Use the child's school spelling list to provide the words for the exercises.
- Large, thick chalk works well for these exercises, especially for children younger than seven.
- If the child has not yet started cursive writing, use the pre-cursive motifs in figure 10.1 instead of words for approximately three weeks, following the same routine described for fine motor exercises. After practicing these pre-cursive motifs for three weeks, the child should be better prepared to begin cursive writing.

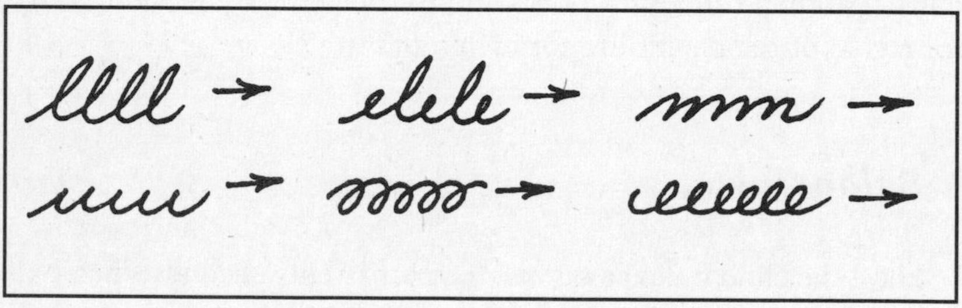

FIGURE 10.1. **Pre-Cursive Motifs**

- For training in cursive writing, teach the letters in the order shown in figure 10.2, based on a combination of ease of production and frequency of use.

1. m, n	*m (m), n (n)*	8. o	*o (o)*
2. e, l	*e, l*	9. q, g	*q, g*
3. i, t	*i, t*	10. f, j	*f, j*
4. c, a	*c (C), a (a)*	11. v, w	*v (v), w (w)*
5. d, p	*d, p*	12. r	*r or r*
6. b, h, k	*b, h, k*	13. y, z	*y (y), z*
7. u, s	*u, s*	14. x	*x*

FIGURE 10.2. **Cursive Letters in Preferred Order of Presentation**

Exercise 1

As you lead the child through this writing exercise, do not allow the child to avoid crossing the midline. Make certain that the child moves the tracing hand across the midline of the body while writing. Many children will consistently and openly avoid crossing the midline. They may tilt or twist the body excessively or turn sideways and walk along the chalkboard while writing the word. Until this task becomes easier for them, these children may have to be held gently but firmly by the shoulders or waist so that they are facing the board squarely.

1. *You* write the model word or row of letters or pre-cursive motif (see figure 10.1) on the chalkboard at the *child's eye level* with letters seven to eight inches high.
2. Have the child stand squarely in front of the chalkboard. The child should be positioned at the middle of the model word, so that as he or she traces the word, the child will have to reach equally to the right and left of the midline of the body and will have to move the tracing hand across the body's midline (see figures 10.3 and 10.4).
3. Smoothly, not painstakingly, have the child trace with a finger over the model word ten times saying each letter while simultaneously tracing. Make certain that the child forms the letters correctly. If

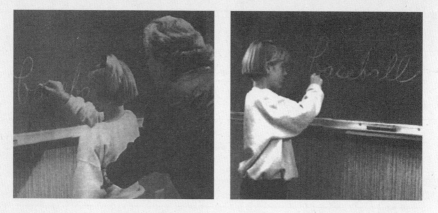

FIGURE 10.3. **Correct Position**   FIGURE 10.4. **Incorrect Position**

the child does not form a letter correctly, have him or her practice tracing a row of that letter before continuing with the model word. Draw arrows indicating the proper direction for letter formation or gently hold the child's hand while he or she is tracing the row of letters.

4. Make certain that the child says the name of the letter simultaneously with the act of tracing it. To be most effective, the spoken sounds must not be ahead of or behind the production of tracing.

5. Then have the child trace over the model word with chalk ten times, repeating the letter while tracing. Pay particular attention to the child's positioning the body correctly, crossing the tracing hand over the midline of the body, and holding the chalk properly. The elbow should be down, not up near the shoulder (see figures 10.5 and 10.6).

   The tracing should be done with expansive, easy motions. The tracing should definitely follow the model, but not with painful, stilted precision.

6. Erase the word and have the child write the word with chalk from memory, saying the name of each letter while simultaneously writing it. All movements should be large arm movements, not cramped small-muscle movements. The child should cross the midline in the reproduction of the word.

7. If the child is unsuccessful in correctly reproducing the word

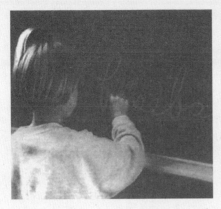 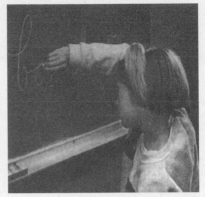

FIGURE 10.5. **Correct Position**   FIGURE 10.6. **Incorrect Position**

from memory, begin again with step #1 and continue in like fashion until the child can write it from memory.

Work for proper sequencing of the letters, movements that are smooth and rhythmical, better formation of the letters, crossing the midline of the body, large-muscle movements, and ease of writing.

Do this exercise five times a week, for approximately 10 minutes a day for three to five weeks.

Exercise 2

Begin this exercise when the child can write the words in Exercise 1 relatively easily and with fairly legible letters.

1. Write a model word in large cursive letters with a pencil or crayon on a large piece of paper, such as butcher paper or wrapping paper.
2. With the paper on a table, have the child trace the word with a finger six or seven times.
3. Then have the child trace the model word with a crayon or odorless Magic Marker six or seven times.
4. Then have the child write the word from memory on another piece of paper.

Do this activity for approximately ten times a day, five days a week, for two to three weeks.

Exercise 3

Following Exercise 2, move on to this writing exercise.

1. Use a piece of paper about the size of typing paper.
2. Repeat the steps in Exercise 2, writing a model word as large as the paper will allow.

Do this exercise for one to two weeks. When the child can write the words legibly and easily, the exercises are completed.

Conclusion

We are as excited today with the STNR program as we were more than thirty years ago, when we first learned of Dr. Miriam L. Bender's work. Through our clinical work, we have been blessed to be able to help make life easier, more productive, and more enjoyable for thousands of people. This book will now enable us to help millions of children and adults.

Some people who read this book may not believe that such a simple solution to such severe problems can be possible. Nevertheless, we have seen this solution work firsthand. Over the years, we have suffered the slings and arrows of other professionals who discount our anecdotal clinic reports or who prefer drug therapy. However, the professionals who have taken the time to listen to the rationale of this program have been delighted to find a new solution to some of the most difficult problems in life.

It is truly impossible to describe the joy of a child who rides a bicycle for the first time after months of falling off, or the face of a child when receiving "The Most Improved Student Award," or the delight of a child who has time to play because homework was accomplished successfully and quickly. It is equally impossible to describe the joy of parents who can now look forward to the time spent with their children, or who can rejoice in their children's free time to play, or who can smile at their children's eagerness to display school papers on the refrigerator. These are the joys that parents and children have shared with us, and now we can share these joys with you.

Reading this book is not enough. You must implement the program—both circumventions and interventions—and share this information with others.

Miriam passed the torch to us. We now pass the torch to you.

God bless you and happy crawling!

P.S. Please send us your success stories for possible future publications.

For further information about our training program and clinic, contact:

Mailing address:
Miriam Bender Achievement Center
c/o Dr. Nancy E. O'Dell
1540 N. Franklin Rd.
Indianapolis, IN 46219
U.S.A.

Phone 1-317-356-0456
e-mail: pcook@uindy.edu
FAX: 1-317-359-4400
web page: www.StoppingADHD.com

To Drug or Not to Drug

To drug or not to drug has become a major issue for parents and educators alike. Many parents feel guilty because they are medicating their ADHD child, and other parents feel guilty because they are *not* medicating their ADHD child. While parents, educators, and physicians are justifiably concerned about the overuse of drugs to treat ADHD, some children probably could not function satisfactorily in the classroom without the initial use of some medication.

Nevertheless, even though medication can sometimes produce beneficial changes in children's behaviors, these medications address only the symptoms, and are *not a cure* for the basic problem. (We have yet to see a child who has been diagnosed as "Ritalin deficient.") It is always better to solve the basic problem, if possible, rather than just contend with the symptoms.

Maturing the STNR will solve a basic problem that causes many, if not all, of the symptoms for at least 75 percent of the individuals diagnosed as ADHD. Unfortunately, until the medical profession becomes aware of and accepts the consequences of an immature STNR, the family physician will continue to be trained in primarily one approach: drug therapy.

Many concerned parents try to research the pros and cons of drug therapy. Turning to the media provides so much information that even a trained professional can hardly keep up with the profusion of books, articles, TV shows, pharmaceutical advertising, and Internet information. The numbers of remedies racing to the market have made knowledge and selection difficult to understand and compare. Educators and parents are in a quandary as to what direction to take. Physicians and psychologists have their hands and their schedules full trying to keep up with the educational and behavioral problems that so many children seem to be experiencing in today's society.

Whether symptoms are proliferating or whether they are being recognized more readily, the diagnoses of behavioral and academic difficulties are dramatically increasing. Parents and educators are demanding a "quick fix" for these children. It is no wonder that the use of drug therapy for ADHD children has escalated to an alarming degree in our "pill popping" world.

A major concern of ours is that parents are very often *not* aware of the potential adverse side effects of these medications. Although new prescriptions come with directions and discussions of the drugs, their purposes, and side effects (often in small print and technical language), many people do not read this information at all. Others stop reading when they encounter difficult chemical names and descriptions. Additionally, some of these drugs are being prescribed "off label," meaning that they are being prescribed for conditions and age groups for which they were not officially tested. Parents who are required to give "informed consent" for medicating their children are often *not* well informed.

We do not say that drug therapy should never be used for ADHD individuals. We do say that drug therapy should be considered last, due to the potential adverse side effects. To our knowledge, every drug has some negative side effect. Physicians and parents/patients must always weigh the benefits against the risks.

Our objective is to present in understandable language some of the negative side effects of ADHD prescription drug treatment. The following list of negative side effects is compiled from ADHD.com, 2003; *Physicians' Desk Reference,* 2003; *Professional's Guide to Patient Drug Facts,* 1995. This is not intended to be a comprehensive list of ADHD medications or negative side effects. Note that not everyone experiences any or all of the negative side effects listed. Some of these side effects occur only rarely. Some of the drugs have additional and varied effects on adults. Note, also, that there can be interactions between one drug and another, and that some foods/drinks can affect the action of a given drug. Be sure to consult your physician and/or pharmacist for advice of such interactions. *Always consult your physician before stopping or changing any aspect of taking any medication.*

Drugs Frequently Prescribed for ADHD and Related Disorders

Stimulants

GENERAL NEGATIVE SIDE EFFECTS

- Loss of appetite
- Sleeplessness (insomnia)
- Weight loss
- Irritability
- Headache
- Nausea
- Stomachaches
- Lack of growth
- Moodiness
- Muscular spasms (tics)

NEGATIVE SIDE EFFECTS FOR SPECIFIC DRUGS

Adderall, Adderall XR (amphetamine)

Rapid heartbeat (tachycardia); fluttering or pounding heartbeat (palpitations); dryness of the mouth; elevation of blood pressure; restlessness; dizziness; sleeplessness; excessive sense of well-being (euphoria); lack of coordination (dyskinesia); anxiety and depression (dysphoria); tremor; headache; increase of muscular spasms (tics); diarrhea; constipation.

Concerta (methylphenidate)
Headache; stomach pain; distorted body image, aversion to food, and extreme weight loss (anorexia); sleeplessness; nervousness; skin rash; hives (urticaria); nausea; vomiting; muscular spasms (tics); allergic reactions; increased blood pressure; abnormal thinking or hallucinations (psychosis).

Cylert (pemoline)
Severe liver dysfunction; convulsive seizures; may lead to Tourette's syndrome (tics); hallucinations; rapid, involuntary, quivering eye movement (nystagmus); mild depression; dizziness; irritability; headache; drowsiness; nausea; stomachache; skin rash; sleeplessness; loss of appetite; weight loss.

Dexedrine (dextroamphetamine)
Rapid heartbeat (tachycardia); fluttering or pounding heartbeat (palpitations); dryness of the mouth; elevation of blood pressure; restlessness; dizziness; sleeplessness (insomnia); excessive sense of well-being (euphoria); lack of coordination (dyskinesia); anxiety and depression (dysphoria); tremor; headache; increase of muscular spasms (tics); diarrhea; constipation; distorted body image, aversion to food, and extreme weight loss (anorexia); hives (urticaria); nausea; irritability; stomach cramps; loss of appetite; nervousness.

Dextrostat (dextroamphetamine sulfate)
Rapid heartbeat (tachycardia); fluttering or pounding heartbeat (palpitations); dryness of the mouth; elevation of blood pressure; restlessness; dizziness; sleeplessness; excessive sense of well-being (euphoria); lack of coordination (dyskinesia); anxiety and depression (dysphoria); tremor; headache; increase of muscular spasms (tics); diarrhea; constipation; distorted body image, aversion to food, and extreme weight loss (anorexia); hives (urticaria).

Focalin (dexmethylphenidate hydrochloride)

Abdominal pain; fever; nausea; twitching; motor or vocal spasms (tics); chest pain (angina); irregular heart rhythm (arrhythmia); fluttering or pounding heartbeat (palpitations); increased or decreased pulse; skin rash; hives (urticaria); dizziness; drowsiness; lack of coordination (dyskinesia); headache; distorted body image, aversion to food, and extreme weight loss (anorexia).

Metadate ER (methylphenidate)

Nervousness; sleeplessness (insomnia); skin rash; hives (urticaria); fever; nausea; dizziness; irregular heartbeat (arrhythmia); fluttering or pounding heartbeat (palpitations); increased or decreased pulse; distorted body image, aversion to food, and extreme weight loss (anorexia); headache; lack of coordination (dyskinesia); blood pressure and pulse changes; rapid heartbeat (tachycardia); chest pain (angina); abdominal pain; weight loss with prolonged use; abnormal liver function.

Methylin ER (methylphenidate)

Nervousness; sleeplessness (insomnia); skin rash; hives (urticaria); fever; joint pain (arthralgia); flaking off skin (exfoliative dermatitis); distorted body image, aversion to food and extreme weight loss (anorexia); dizziness; nausea; fluttering or pounding heartbeat (palpitations); headache; lack of coordination (dyskinesia); drowsiness; blood pressure and pulse changes; rapid heartbeat (tachycardia); chest pain (angina); irregular heartbeat (arrhythmia); abdominal pain; weight loss during prolonged use; loss of appetite.

Ritalin, Ritalin SR (methylphenidate)

Loss of appetite; stomach pain; weight loss with prolonged use; sleeplessness (insomnia); increased heart rate; rash; hives (urticaria); fever; joint pain; peeling skin; redness; nervousness; headache; irregular heartbeat (arrhythmia); fluttering or pounding heartbeat (palpitations); chest pain (angina); joint pain (arthralgia); distorted body image, aversion to food, and extreme weight loss (anorexia); nausea;

dizziness; headache; lack of coordination (dyskinesia); drowsiness; changes in blood pressure and pulse; rapid heartbeat (tachycardia).

Ritalin LA (methylphenidate)

Nervousness; stomach pain; sleeplessness (insomnia); decreased appetite; nausea; vomiting; dizziness; muscular spasms (tics); allergic reactions; increased blood pressure; abnormal thinking or hallucinations (psychosis); blurred vision (this can be the sign of a serious problem); slower growth.

Non-stimulants

General Negative Side Effects
- Upset stomach
- Decreased appetite
- Nausea and vomiting
- Dizziness
- Tiredness
- Mood swings

Negative Side Effects for Specific Drugs

Strattera (atomoxetine HCl)

Indigestion (dyspepsia); nausea; vomiting; fatigue; decreased appetite; mood swings; possible stunted growth; can increase blood pressure and heart rate; pulse and blood pressure should be monitored at baseline (beginning), after each dose increase, and periodically thereafter.

Antihypertensives

General Negative Side Effects
- Drowsiness
- Dry mouth
- Constipation

Negative Side Effects for Specific Drugs

Catapres (clonidine)

Constipation; nausea; dry mouth; vomiting; decreased appetite; depression; nightmares; headache; nervousness; weakness; sleep problems; drowsiness; tingling or burning of hands and feet; drop in blood pressure upon standing, which may cause dizziness, fainting, and blurred vision (orthostatic hypotension); changes in heart rate; fluttering or pounding heartbeat (palpitations); weakness and shortness of breath caused by inadequate blood circulation (congestive heart failure); rash; hives (urticaria); hair thinning (alopecia).

Tenex (guanfacine)

Constipation; nausea; vomiting; stomachache; diarrhea; memory loss; confusion; dizziness; headache; sedation; severe weakness; sleeplessness (insomnia); numbness or tingling of the hands or feet; depression; slow pulse; irregular heartbeat (arrhythmia); chest pain (angina); shortness of breath; runny nose; itching; inflammation of skin; sweating; dry mouth; drowsiness; gas pains; loss of appetite; fatigue; stuffy nose (nasal congestion); skin rash; swelling of the hands or feet (edema); blurred vision; yellowing of eyes or skin (jaundice).

Antidepressants

General Negative Side Effects

- Headache
- Sleeplessness (insomnia)
- Weight loss
- Nervousness
- Constipation or diarrhea

In March 2004, the Food and Drug Administration (FDA) asked the drug manufacturers to put a stronger warning on ten antidepressants, concerning signs of suicidal thoughts: Celexa, Effexor,

Lexapro, Luvox, Paxil, Prozac, Remeron, Serzone, Wellbutrin, Zoloft. (*Indianapolis Star* 2004)

Negative Side Effects for Specific Drugs

Celexa (citalopram hydrobromide)

Suicidal thoughts; dry mouth; drowsiness (somnolence); coughing; rash; nausea; severe itching (pruritis); taste changes; excessive passage of urine (polyuria).

Effexor (venlafaxine)

Suicidal thoughts; nausea; constipation; distorted body image, aversion to food and extreme weight loss (anorexia); diarrhea; vomiting; indigestion; gas; difficulty swallowing; belching; drowsiness; sleeplessness (insomnia); dizziness; nervousness; feeling of being in whirling surroundings (vertigo); dry mouth; anxiety; trembling (tremor); nightmares; confusion; increased blood pressure; increased heart rate; severe headache (migraine); difficulty breathing; itching; rash; sweating; weakness (asthenia).

Elavil (amitriptyline)

Nausea; vomiting; indigestion; constipation; loss of appetite; increased appetite; upset stomach and cramps; diarrhea; gas; seizures; anxiety; nervousness; muscle spasms or tremors; drowsiness; sleep disturbances; nightmares; fatigue; headache; severe headache (migraine); memory loss; dizziness; abnormal thinking or hallucinations (psychosis); unusually high body temperature (hyperthermia); restlessness; panic; depression; yawning; irritability; rapid heartbeat (tachycardia); fluttering or pounding heartbeat (palpitations); drop in blood pressure upon standing, which may cause dizziness, fainting, and blurred vision (orthostatic hypotension); increased or decreased blood pressure; irregular heartbeat (arrhythmia); urinary problems; rash; sensitivity to light (photosensitivity); dry mouth; blurred vision; weight changes; chills; nose bleeds; excessive thirst; tingling or burning of the arms and legs (paresthesia); itching.

Lexapro (escitalopram oxalate)

Suicidal thoughts; drowsiness (somnolence); sleeplessness (insomnia); diarrhea; dry mouth; dizziness; sweating; constipation; fatigue; indigestion; nausea.

Luvox (fluvoxamine)

Suicidal thoughts; nausea; drowsiness; dizziness; diarrhea; trouble sleeping; constipation; upset stomach; dry mouth; vomiting; loss of appetite; unusual or severe mental/mood changes; sweating or reddening; unusual fatigue; uncontrolled trembling; blurred vision; rapid heartbeat (tachycardia); tingling or numbness of the hands or feet; muscle pain; trouble swallowing; seizures; easy bruising or bleeding.

Norpramin (desipramine)

Nausea; vomiting; indigestion; constipation; loss of appetite; increased appetite; upset stomach and cramps; diarrhea; gas; seizures; anxiety; nervousness; muscle spasms or tremors; drowsiness; sleep disturbances; nightmares; fatigue; headache; severe headache (migraine); memory loss; dizziness; abnormal thinking or hallucinations (psychosis); unusually high body temperature (hyperthermia); restlessness; panic; depression; yawning; irritability; rapid heartbeat (tachycardia); fluttering or pounding heartbeat (palpitations); drop in blood pressure upon standing, which may cause dizziness, fainting, blurred vision (orthostatic hypotension); increased or decreased blood pressure; irregular heartbeat (arrhythmia); urinary problems; rash; sensitivity to light (photosensitivity); dry mouth; blurred vision; weight changes; chills; nose bleeds; excessive thirst; tingling or burning of the arms and legs (paresthesia); itching.

Pamelor (nortriptyline)

Nausea; vomiting; indigestion; constipation; loss of appetite; increased appetite; upset stomach and cramps; diarrhea; gas; seizures; anxiety; nervousness; muscle spasms or tremors; drowsiness; sleep disturbances; nightmares; fatigue; headache; severe headache (migraine); memory loss; dizziness; abnormal thinking or hallucinations (psychosis); unusually high body temperature (hyperthermia);

restlessness; panic; depression; yawning; irritability; rapid heartbeat (tachycardia); fluttering or pounding heartbeat (palpitations); drop in blood pressure upon standing, which may cause dizziness, fainting, and blurred vision (orthostatic hypotension); increased or decreased blood pressure; irregular heartbeat (arrhythmia); urinary problems; rash; sensitivity to light (photosensitivity); dry mouth; blurred vision; weight changes; chills; nose bleeds; excessive thirst; tingling or burning of the arms and legs (paresthesia); itching.

Paxil (paroxetine)

Suicidal thoughts; nausea; diarrhea; vomiting; stomach pain; constipation; gas; indigestion; changes in appetite; drowsiness; sleeplessness (insomnia); being upset (agitation); anxiety; headache; dizziness; nervousness; twitching; inability to concentrate; depression; feeling of being in whirling surroundings (vertigo); fluttering or pounding heartbeat (palpitations); high blood pressure (hypertension); yawning; sore throat; cough; reddening; sweating; rash; severe itching (pruritus); dry mouth; fever; back pain; rapid heartbeat (tachycardia); drop in blood pressure upon standing, which may cause dizziness, fainting, and blurred vision (orthostatic hypotension); urinary disorders; chills; fluid retention (edema); weight changes; joint pain (arthralgia); emotional instability; chronic ringing or buzzing in the ears (tinnitus).

Prozac (fluoxetine)

Suicidal thoughts; stomach upset; indigestion; vomiting; nausea; appetite changes; distorted body image, aversion to food, and extreme weight loss (anorexia); diarrhea; constipation; gas; blood in stools or vomit; trembling (tremor); anxiety; dizziness; light-headedness; drowsiness; headache; sleeplessness (insomnia); fatigue; decreased concentration; abnormal dreams or thinking; loss of memory; confusion; being upset (agitation); twitching; psychological disturbances; fluttering or pounding heartbeat (palpitations); chest pain (angina); hot flashes; reddening; upper respiratory tract infections; cough; yawning; painful or difficult breathing; rash; hives (urticaria); severe itching (pruritus); sweating; acne; urinary and reproductive tract dysfunction; fever; fluid retention (edema); joint pain (arthralgia); dry mouth; vision disturbances; chronic ringing or buzzing in the ears (tinnitus); chills; muscle cramps; weight changes; high blood pressure (hypertension); emotional instability; ear pain.

Remeron (mirtazapine)

Suicidal thoughts; drowsiness (somnolence); dry mouth; impairment of psychomotor performance; increased appetite; weight gain; constipation; abdominal pain; dizziness; high blood pressure (hypertension); thirst; vomiting; abnormal weakness or fatigue (myasthenia); joint pain (arthralgia); partial loss of the sense of touch or feeling (hypesthesia); lack of interest or concern (apathy); depression; cough; sinusitis; severe itching (pruritus); urinary tract infection.

Serzone (nefazodone hydrochloride)

Suicidal thoughts; drowsiness (somnolence); dry mouth; nausea; dizziness; constipation; weakness (asthenia); light-headedness; blurred vision; confusion; abnormal vision.

Tofranil (imipramine)

Nausea; vomiting; indigestion; constipation; loss of appetite; increased appetite; upset stomach and cramps; diarrhea; gas; seizures; anxiety; nervousness; muscle spasms or tremors; drowsiness; sleep disturbances; nightmares; fatigue; headache; severe headache (migraine); memory loss; dizziness; abnormal thinking or hallucinations (psychosis); unusually high body temperature (hyperthermia); restlessness; panic; depression; yawning; irritability; rapid heartbeat (tachycardia); fluttering or pounding heartbeat (palpitations); drop in blood pressure upon standing, which may cause dizziness, fainting, and blurred vision (orthostatic hypotension); increased or decreased blood pressure; irregular heartbeat (arrhythmia); urinary problems; rash; sensitivity to light (photosensitivity); dry mouth; blurred vision; weight changes; chills; nose bleeds; excessive thirst; tingling or burning of the arms and legs (paresthesia); itching.

Wellbutrin (bupropion)

Suicidal thoughts; trembling (tremor); drooling; muscle stiffness; rigidity; shuffling walk; incoordination (ataxia); nausea; vomiting; diarrhea; constipation; indigestion; changes in appetite; seizures; dizziness; muscle spasms; delusions; mood or personality changes; exaggerated sense of well-being (euphoria); confusion; being upset (agitation); hostility; disturbed concentration; restlessness; sleep disturbances; fatigue; headache; fluttering or pounding heartbeat (palpitations); irregular heartbeat (arrhythmia); rapid heartbeat (tachycardia); changes in blood pressure; rash; severe itching (pruritus); excessive sweating; dry mouth; changes in taste; blurred vision; hearing problems; frequent urination; urinary retention; fever; chills; weight loss or gain; fainting; arthritis; high blood pressure (hypertension); fluid retention (edema); a sudden twitching of muscles (myclonus); lack of coordination (dyskinesia); hallucinations; depression; exaggerated high spirits (mania); flu-like symptoms; joint pain (arthralgia).

Zoloft (sertraline)

Suicidal thoughts; nausea; vomiting; diarrhea; indigestion; constipation; stomachache; gas; appetite changes; headache; dizziness; trembling (tremor); twitching; fatigue; nervousness; anxiety; drowsiness; being upset (agitation); sleeplessness (insomnia); decreased concentration; fluttering or pounding heartbeat (palpitations); chest pain (angina); dry mouth; fever; thirst; runny nose; sore throat; chronic ringing or buzzing in the ears (tinnitus); changes in taste; back pain; sweating; hot flashes; rash; yawning; hyperactivity (hyperkinesis); burst blood vessels in the skin (purpura); weight decrease; exaggerated high spirits (mania); abnormal thinking; nose bleed (epistaxis); extreme muscular tension (hypertonia); yawning.

Anticonvulsants

GENERAL NEGATIVE SIDE EFFECTS
- Headache
- Sleeplessness (insomnia)

- Weight loss
- Decreased appetite
- Trembling (tremor)
- Hair loss (alopecia)
- Feeling of being in whirling surroundings (vertigo)

NEGATIVE SIDE EFFECTS FOR SPECIFIC DRUGS

Depakote (divalproex sodium)

(Children under two years: considerable increased risk of fatal liver damage); severe threat of fatal liver damage; changes in appetite; nausea; vomiting; stomach cramps; indigestion; diarrhea; constipation; weakness; tiredness; clumsiness; drowsiness; behavior changes; depression; headache; yellowing of skin or eyes (jaundice); burst blood vessels in the skin (purpura); rash; swelling of the face, hands, and feet (edema); double vision; spots before the eyes; unusual eye movements; weight gain or loss; hair loss (alopecia).

Tegretol (carbamazepine)

Abnormal liver and kidney function tests; weakness and shortness of breath caused by inadequate blood circulation (congestive heart failure); nausea; vomiting; upset stomach; stomachache; diarrhea; constipation; pale stools; appetite loss; drowsiness; dizziness; incoordination; headache; confusion; mood changes; behavior changes especially in children; slurred speech; hallucinations; depression; fatigue; difficulty breathing; pneumonia; yellowing of skin or eyes (jaundice); easy bruising or bleeding; rash; hives (urticaria); sensitivity to sunlight (photosensitivity); sweating; hair loss (alopecia); aggravation of the condition of lupus; double vision; blurred vision; red itchy eyes; urinary frequency; urinary retention; dark urine; fainting; fever; chills; sore throat; ulcers in the mouth; dry mouth; inflammation of the mouth or tongue; muscle and joint aches (arthralgia); leg cramps; swelling of legs or ankles (edema); swollen glands; numbness in hands or feet; chronic ringing or buzzing in ears (tinnitus); abnormal sensitivity to sounds; severe itching (pruritus).

Antianxiety medications

General Negative Side Effects
- Constipation or diarrhea
- Headache
- Loss of memory
- Nausea, vomiting
- Clumsiness
- A "hangover" effect
- Difficulty sleeping, nightmares
- Dizziness
- Drowsiness
- Unsteadiness

Negative Side Effects for Specific Drugs

Ativan (lorazepam)
Abnormal liver function; stomach upset; constipation; diarrhea; nausea; change in appetite; vomiting; confusion; hallucinations; depression; nervousness; behavior changes; memory loss; drowsiness; fatigue; dizziness; feeling of being in whirling surroundings (vertigo); lack of interest or concern (apathy); exaggerated sense of well-being (euphoria); restlessness; crying; sleep disturbances; incoordination; vivid dreams; headache; seizures; weakness; unsteadiness; irregular heartbeat (arrhythmia); changes in blood pressure; fluttering or pounding heartbeat (palpitations); slow pulse; hives (urticaria); severe itching (pruritus); rash; hair loss (alopecia); excessive hair growth; yellowing of skin or eyes (jaundice); double vision; blurred vision; decreased hearing; hearing disturbances; nasal congestion; slurred speech; loss of voice; lack of urinary control; dry mouth; difficulty swallowing; sore throat; hiccups; fever; chills; balance problems; trembling (tremor); breathing problems; ankle and facial swelling (edema); "glassy-eyed" appearance; increased salivation; sore gums;

coated tongue; excessive sweating; joint pain (arthralgia); weight gain or loss; lack of body fluid (dehydration); swollen lymph nodes; fainting; unusual bleeding or bruising.

BuSpar (buspirone)

Dizziness; nausea; headache; nervousness; light-headedness; stomach upset; diarrhea; constipation; vomiting; gas; changes in appetite; salivation; irritable colon; rectal bleeding; dream disturbances; drowsiness; fatigue; weakness; sleeplessness (insomnia); decreased concentration; anger; confusion; depression; numbness; incoordination; trembling (tremor); chest pain (angina); rapid heartbeat (tachycardia); changes in blood pressure; fluttering or pounding heartbeat (palpitations); abnormally fast or deep breathing (hyperventilation); shortness of breath; rash; severe itching (pruritus); reddening; easy bruising; hair loss (alopecia); dry skin; blisters; sweating; clamminess; chronic ringing or buzzing in the ears (tinnitus); sore throat; blurred vision; nasal congestion; redness and itching of the eyes; changes in taste and smell; dry mouth; weight gain or loss; fever; urinary problems; muscle spasms; joint pain (arthralgia); fluid retention (edema); twitching.

Antipsychotics

GENERAL NEGATIVE SIDE EFFECTS

- Drowsiness
- Nausea
- Muscle stiffness
- Difficulty swallowing

NEGATIVE SIDE EFFECTS FOR SPECIFIC DRUGS

Risperdal (risperidone)

Dizziness; drowsiness; nausea; increased dreaming; nervousness; loss of appetite; dry mouth; fatigue; weight gain; vision changes; increased sleep duration; sleeplessness (insomnia); irregular heartbeat (arrhythmia); fluttering or pounding heartbeat (palpitations); rapid heartbeat (tachycardia); itching; difficulty moving; muscle stiffness; twitching; sweating; drooling; trembling (tremor); difficulty swallowing; mental confusion; seizures; distorted body image, aversion to food and extreme weight loss (anorexia); sensitivity to light (photosensitivity).

Zyprexa (olanzapine)

Stomach pain; nausea; dizziness; rapid heartbeat (tachycardia); dry mouth; constipation; weight changes; ankles and legs swelling (edema); drowsiness; being upset (agitation); restlessness; pink urine; fever; confusion; muscle stiffness; dental pain; flu-like symptoms; intentional injury and suicide attempt; low blood pressure (hypotension); increased salivation and thirst; low white blood cell count; twitching; joint stiffness; abnormal dreams; exaggerated sense of well-being (euphoria); difficulty breathing (dyspnea); sweating; inflammation of the eyelid (conjunctivitis); may infrequently make blood sugar level rise; difficulty swallowing.

Anti-Mania Medication

Eskalith (lithium carbonate)

Tiredness; increased thirst; frequent urination; weight gain; trembling of the hands (tremor); diarrhea; vomiting; drowsiness; fever; unsteady walking; fainting; confusion; slurred speech; rapid heartbeat (tachycardia); irregular heartbeat (arrhythmia); nausea; muscular weakness; lack of coordination; giddiness; chronic ringing or buzzing in the ears (tinnitus); blurred vision; large output of diluted urine; distorted body image, aversion to food and extreme weight loss (anorexia); excess sugar in the urine (glycosuria); loss of hair (alopecia); blurred vision.

Abridged Glossary of Medical Terms

agitation: A state of being upset.

alopecia: Hair thinning or hair loss.

angina: Chest pain.

anorexia: Distorted body image, aversion to food, and extreme weight loss.

apathy: Lack of interest or concern.

arrhythmia: Irregular heartbeat.

arthralgia: Joint pain.

asthenia: Weakness.

ataxia: Incoordination.

congestive heart failure: Weakness and shortness of breath caused by inadequate blood circulation.

conjunctivitis: Inflammation of the eyelid.

dehydration: Lack of body fluid.

dyskinesia: Lack of coordination.

dyspepsia: Indigestion.

dysphoria: Anxiety and depression.

dyspnea: Difficulty breathing.

edema: Fluid retention.

epistaxis: Nose bleeding.

euphoria: Exaggerated sense of well-being.

exfoliative dermatitis: Flaking of skin.

glycosuria: Excess sugar in the urine.

hypertension: High blood pressure.

hyperthermia: Unusually high body temperature.

hypertonia: Extreme muscular tension.

hyperventilation: Abnormally fast and deep breathing.

hypesthesia: Partial loss of the sense of touch or feeling.

insomnia: Sleeplessness.

mania: Exaggerated high spirits.

migraine: Severe headache.

myasthesia: Abnormal muscular weakness or fatigue.

myclonus: A sudden twitching of muscles.

nystagmus: Rapid, involuntary, quivering eye movement.

orthostatic hypotension: Drop in blood pressure upon standing—which may cause dizziness, fainting, blurred vision.

palpitations: Fluttering or pounding heartbeat.

paresthesia: Burning or tingling of skin.

photosensitivity: Sensitivity to light.

polyuria: Excessive passage of urine.

pruritus: Severe itching.

psychosis: Abnormal thinking or hallucinations.

purpura: Burst blood vessels in the skin.

somnolence: Drowsiness.

tachycardia: Rapid heartbeat.

tics: Muscular spasms.

tinnitus: Chronic ringing or buzzing in the ears.

tremor: Trembling.

urticaria: Hives.

vertigo: Feeling of being in whirling surroundings.

Questions and Answers

Since the publication of the first edition of our book in 1997, we have received letters, phone calls, and e-mails from all over the world—from the United States, Australia, Austria, West Indies, Canada, South America, England, Finland, Germany, Israel, Mexico, Norway, Scotland, Singapore, South Africa, Sweden, and Taiwan. Here are the most frequently asked questions, with our responses:

Do these STNR exercises really work?
Absolutely, if they are done properly.

What is ADD/ADHD called now? I'm confused with all the alphabet soups.
Your confusion is understandable. ADHD is now the most widely used term. It includes difficulties with both attention and/or hyperactivity. It is usually written as attention-deficit/hyperactivity disorder.

Why isn't this approach to remediation of ADHD better known?
The rule of thumb for information reaching the public from initial research is at least twenty-five years. Although we have been doing this work for over thirty years, the medical profession, in general, has not yet embraced this remedial approach.

Why hasn't the medical community been more open to this approach?

This research came through education, rather than through medicine, and the medical community tends to be reluctant to accept therapies outside their own discipline. Because of this tunnel vision, most physicians have not even heard of the immature STNR in connection with ADHD. (Remember that William Harvey was laughed at by the medical profession when he said that blood ran in vessels; also, physicians did not believe Pasteur when he presented his theory about germs.) Fortunately, alternative/complementary approaches are beginning to be more readily accepted by the medical community, primarily because of a groundswell of public demand.

I'm doing the STNR exercises with our five-year-old, but now we also have a seven-month-old baby who is not even rocking, let alone crawling. Is there anything I can do to help this baby start rocking so that she will crawl?

Try to get your baby into the Cat Sit Position (p. 20). Then kneel beside her and gently rock her up into the Box Position (p. 21) and then back down into the Cat Sit Position. You will have to provide the motion for the baby. Do this several times. DO NOT use any physical pressure on the baby. Do this several times a day for a couple of weeks. If she doesn't start voluntarily rocking and/or crawling, don't worry. You can correct this reflex problem when she is five years old. DO NOT try to force rocking or crawling.

My family is constantly holding on to my seven-month-old baby's hands, trying to get her to walk. What can I do?

Lovingly (gently) smack your family's collective hands and tell them to let go and let that baby crawl! Tell them how important it is for a baby to crawl extensively for at least six months, and have them read our book.

My child is four years old. Can we do the STNR exercises?

No. You need to wait until your child is five years old. Important development (neurological, physical, physiological, etc.) occurs between the ages of four and five that will enable the child to be better able to do the STNR exercises. Until then, do not make the child sit for long periods of time. Follow our book's recommendations for circumventions.

My child is only three years old, so I know I can't start the STNR exercise program, but her activity level is driving me crazy. Any other suggestions?

Follow our book's recommendations for circumventions. Consider dietary changes, specifically the elimination of sugar and dairy products, and the possibility of low blood sugar (hypoglycemia). Here are three of the many good books about nutrition and ADHD on the market: *Prescription for Nutritional Healing*, by P. and J. Balch; *Help for the Hyperactive Child*, by W. Crook; *12 Effective Ways to Help Your ADD/ADHD Child*, by L. Stevens.

My nine-month-old baby isn't crawling and is trying to stand up and walk around the room, holding on to furniture. How do I make him crawl?

Do not, under any circumstances, try to force a baby to crawl. Encourage him to crawl by giving ample opportunity and space in which to crawl and by getting down on the floor with him and encouraging him to follow your example of crawling. You can gently put him in the Cat Sit Position (see page 20) and rock him gently back and forth. *Do not* use any physical pressure on him. If the baby fights all these attempts to encourage crawling, wait until he is five years old to do the STNR exercises.

We received a baby walker at a shower. What should we do?

Return it to the store if you can, or use it as a flowerpot. *Do not* put your baby in a walker, Johnny jump up, doorway swing, or anything else that prohibits crawling. Use playpens sparingly or only when absolutely necessary.

My friend knew not to give me a walker for my ten-month-old baby. Instead she gave me a toy grocery cart for my baby to stand behind and push. Is this okay to use?

These lightweight, stand-up-behind-and-push playthings are merely the twenty-first century's version of baby walkers. *Do not* use them until your baby has crawled properly for at least six months and is walking independently well.

Is there an age that's too old to benefit from the STNR exercises?

No age is too old to benefit from the STNR exercises. So far, the oldest person we have worked with was seventy-seven. She said she was tired of being uncomfortable all her life. After doing the STNR exercises, she really appreciated being able to sit more comfortably at church and when playing games with her great-grandchildren.

Can the problems from the STNR be inherited?

It has been our observation that an immature STNR often runs in families. You inherit your hair color, eye color, bone structure, etc.; reflexes are also inherited.

Can environmental factors cause an immature STNR?

Yes. If a baby's crawling is prohibited or significantly restricted, the STNR will remain immature (at an interfering level). Overuse of playpens, limited crawling space, leg casts, or any environmental situation that interferes with enough (at least six months) and proper crawling will lead to an immature STNR.

My child didn't crawl and has all the STNR symptoms. Can't he just outgrow these problems?

No. If a baby does not crawl enough and properly, the STNR will remain immature unless the individual has special help to mature it.

My son had many immature STNR symptoms, but through years of tremendous effort in sports, has become much better coordinated than he was. Can large muscle activity mature the STNR? He still has trouble writing legibly.

Many years of large muscle (gross motor) activity can help, but vestiges of the STNR will always remain unless directly treated. See chapter 2.

My child does not have all the symptoms listed in the book, but he has a terrible time with sports. He walked at nine months. Could he have STNR?

Yes, he could have an immature STNR, even though it is unlikely that any individual will have all of the symptoms. Frequently a child will display only one or two of the symptoms. However, any individual who did not crawl for at least six months and/or properly will be bothered in some way by an immature STNR.

Could maturing the STNR adversely affect some of the good things that seem to come from being "this way"? Good things like hyperactivity channeled into energy to have a successful business or the extra energy our son has on the baseball field (he can't sit on the bench, but is an excellent batter).

Maturing the STNR will significantly improve total coordination and control. While some seemingly positive explosive aspects of the immature reflex may be lost, the overall improvement in ease, comfort, control, coordination, and organization will more than make up for it. We want the child to control the body, not the body to control the child.

My child's handwriting looks like chicken scratch, but he seems to have no trouble with some of the things your book says he should have trouble with. He did the "army crawl" for four months and then walked. Does he have STNR?

An individual who did not crawl for at least six months and/or properly will be bothered in some way by an immature STNR. However, with great effort and energy, some STNR children can become competent at a number of tasks. Remember, too, that some activities seem to "bypass" the immature reflex, and a child can seem to be excelling in a sport, for example, but be good at only one aspect, e.g., seemingly a good swimmer, but capable at only a specific stroke. See the section in the book on sports.

Can the STNR cause children to have difficulty getting along with siblings?

Yes. The frustration and fatigue caused by an immature STNR can lead to a "short fuse," and heightened aggression in many cases. Children can frequently get along at home *or* at school, but don't have the energy to get along both places. They cannot maintain working ten times harder constantly. Siblings (and others) become annoyed right back because they don't realize the STNR child is having to work so hard.

How do we get a teenager to do the exercises?

If a child is old enough to realize the difficulties s/he is having, explain the significant benefits that will occur from doing these exercises, e.g., writing will be easier, sitting still will be more comfortable, etc. We are great believers in positive reinforcement. Everybody loves rewards, and you are rewarding the child for cooperating in a very difficult task. Daily exercises can earn daily stickers or tokens to be exchanged for a designated reward down the line. See chapter 9, "The STNR Exercises: General Directions."

Do children with an immature STNR frequently display noisemaking, nervous tics, and other negative mannerisms?

Yes. Many children with an immature STNR often have nervous tics, make excessive and/or inappropriate noises, or display other negative mannerisms. Frequently these mannerisms significantly diminish or totally disappear upon the individual's successful completion of the STNR exercises.

Can an autistic child benefit from the STNR exercises?

Any individual who has not crawled for at least six months and properly can benefit from doing the STNR exercises. (It is our understanding that most autistic children do not crawl for at least six months and/or properly.)

Are the ATNR (asymmetric tonic neck reflex) and the STNR (symmetric tonic neck reflex) the same thing?

No. The ATNR, commonly referred to as the fencing reflex (because of the position of the baby's arms) appears earlier than the STNR in the infant's development.

Do we need to do exercises to mature the ATNR as well as the STNR?

It has been our experience that the STNR exercises mature not only the STNR, but also the ATNR.

Can parents do the exercises with their children, or do we need a PT (physical therapist) or an OT (occupational therapist)?

The STNR exercises are designed for nonprofessionals to be able to implement the program successfully. In over thirty years of clinic work, we have successfully trained parents, teachers, grandparents, siblings, other relatives, neighbors, and friends to be the "crawling therapists." Of course, OTs and PTs can certainly implement these exercises, but their higher level of expertise is not required for the daily implementation of the program. Because of their professional background, we would love to have OTs and PTs receive certification in the STNR exercise program, acting as directors of additional clinics of the Miriam Bender Achievement Center around the world.

Will we ever have to do these exercises again once we have finished the program?

No. Once the STNR reflex is matured, it stays matured, just as when a baby naturally crawls long enough and properly. (However, we theorize the possibility that a specific neurological trauma such as a stroke or brain injury from an accident might reestablish the STNR's interfering effects.)

We had done the exercises for three months. And then, because of unforeseen circumstances, we had to stop doing them for a month. Do we have to start from the beginning?

No, don't start over from the very beginning. The individual will retain whatever had been gained at the point of interruption. Pick up where you left off. (S/he may be a little out of rhythm for a few days.) Be sure that your calendar time is at least a full eight months of doing the STNR exercises, and not just eight months from the time you began (to account for any interruptions). Remember that smooth and satisfactory performance at each stage of the STNR program is more important than tallying eight months on the calendar.

Can we split the exercises up into two sessions a day, rather than doing them all at once?

Yes, the STNR exercises can be split into two or three smaller sessions a day if that works better into the family's schedule or is easier for the child (especially for a younger child).

My child is throwing his head way back when he does the exercises. Is that necessary?

No. It is not necessary to hyper-extend the neck (throw the head way back). Nevertheless, some children seem to have to exaggerate the head raising in order to be aware that the head is up. (See figures 9.1 through 9.3.)

My child says his neck hurts when he's doing the exercises. Am I doing something wrong, or will the pain go away?

Most children experience some discomfort in their necks when first doing the STNR exercises. It's possible that you are increasing their discomfort if you are giving too much resistance. (We would prefer that the crawling therapist provide too little resistance rather than too much.) Provide neck rubs and occasional breaks during the STNR exercises. This neck pain (notice we avoid the phrase "pain in the neck") usually subsides within two to three months.

After three months of doing the STNR exercises, my child still says his neck hurts when he's crawling. What should I do?

If a child's neck still hurts three months into the STNR exercise program, we highly recommend taking that child to a chiropractor or an osteopath for proper body alignment. Many STNR children develop misalignment of their bodies because of frequent falling due to the discoordination and clumsiness caused by the immature STNR. Once the child's body is properly aligned, the head can be more easily raised with less discomfort while doing the STNR exercises.

My child wants to crawl with his hands curled up in fists or with them turned out. Is this all right?

In the beginning, we don't want you to be fussing at the child about everything. The head position is always the most important concern. Initially, follow the directions for the correct positioning, figure 9.1. *One time a trip,* you may tell the child to flatten his hands, pointing the fingers straight ahead. If you remind him about too many things at the same time, he will just "overload" and tune you out. When the child is ready for modifications (see figure 9.26), after gaining control of the head position, then you may more directly address the hand position.

My child wants to crawl with her eyes shut. Is that okay?

No. It is important that the child try to watch a target at her eye level as much as possible throughout the exercises.

My child's head is up, but I can tell he's looking around the room. Is that all right?

No. It is important that the child try to watch a target at his eye level as much as possible. Watching the target will help develop visual focusing and attention. Many STNR children have inadequate eye control; it has been our experience that eye control improves significantly after completing the STNR exercises while watching a target. If you can, put a TV at the end of the crawling runway and consider using a favorite TV show or movie as the target.

My child wants to have a running conversation while doing the exercises. Is that all right?

If the child's talking *does not interfere* with the performance, then talk away. If the crawling performance deteriorates when the child is talking, then conversation needs to be curtailed.

My child says I am pushing/pulling too hard. It seems like I am barely touching him. How can I know how much resistance to use?

Trust the child. The child is the *only* one who knows if the resistance is too much or too little. You must not push/pull too hard. It is always better to give too little resistance than too much.

My child says it hurts when I am pushing/pulling during the exercises. Should I put my hands in a different spot?

Slight variation of your hand positioning is acceptable so long as the basic performance of the exercise is not significantly altered. If a slight change in hand position doesn't solve the problem, see the section "Alternative Positions."

I am tired of saying "Pull," and "Push." My child knows the routine. Do I have to keep saying these words?

Yes. It is essential to continue giving the verbal directions. There is significant benefit to the child in receiving simultaneous, multisensory information: auditory, tactile, and kinesthetic (muscular). It is important that the verbal command and the kinesthetic tug or nudge occur exactly at the same time. Do not let the child move until you have given the verbal direction. We theorize that requiring the child to wait for the verbal command promotes the establishment of neurological structures that will allow the child to gain control over impulsive actions.

What if my child doesn't seem ready for the next exercise, and/or it's too hard for her?

Maintain the program that she is successful with until she can reasonably succeed with the next exercise. Do not force her to advance prematurely.

When my child is doing the exercises, he is moving the arm
and leg on the same side of his body, instead of in an alternating fashion. Should I force an alternating pattern on him?

No, do not force any particular pattern on him. Almost every
child starts out crawling by moving the arm and leg on the same side
(ipsilateral). Most children will automatically work into the alternate movement pattern (reciprocal) in their own sweet time, or else
they will develop a highly coordinated ipsilateral pattern. (One of
our clients lovingly calls her daughter "Ipsi.") However, *in forward
crawling only,* children can often be eased into a reciprocal pattern.
They are usually ready for such a modification when they are ready
for Crawling III. See chapter 9, "Modifications for Crawling II."

Sometimes my child moves both hands when he moves one
leg, mostly when crawling backward. Is this all right?

No, the child should not move both hands at the same time. Encourage the child to move either hand with one leg. Do not try to
force a specific arm/leg pattern on the child. The child's body will
work it out. A reciprocal pattern is not necessary for backward crawling. See the previous answer.

If we do the crawling exercises seven days a week, instead of
five days, can we be finished sooner?

Possibly, but in over thirty years of implementing this program, we
have never had anybody maintain crawling seven days a week for an
extended period of time. Having two days off a week gives everybody
a breather and also the opportunity to make up any unexpected lapse
in the STNR exercise routine. Remember that a smooth and satisfactory performance at each stage of the STNR program is more important than tallying eight months on the calendar.

I want to do the exercise program with my child, but I cannot be on my knees to crawl. What can I do?

See "Alternative Positions," or come to our clinic, where we can
personally guide you.

A problem I have is that my house is hardwood throughout and there isn't really an area to put down a carpet remnant. For the crawling surface, could a grassy area substitute for a carpeted floor?

You need a straight area that is ideally twenty feet long (minimum of fifteen feet). The area needs to be just wider than your body, so hallways are excellent, or you can crawl from one room through a doorway into another room. You *must* protect your knees—with "store-bought" knee pads (e.g., those for wrestlers or volleyball players)—or homemade knee pads. If the only straight area long enough is outside, use a carpet remnant on the ground, and be sure to protect your knees, legs, and feet.

Our child is on medication, and we have just started the exercise program. Should we stop the medication?

We cannot professionally tell you to stop using the ADHD medication, especially if your child seems to be benefiting from it. Fortunately, it has been our experience that once the STNR has been matured through the exercise program, most children can stop their ADHD medications and perform even better than when they were on them. Many parents use the physician-recommended summer months to stop the ADHD medications. *Always* consult your physician for the proper procedure if you choose to stop or change the medications, as some should be discontinued gradually, rather than all at once.

Are there different STNR exercises for an adult?

The STNR exercises are the same for adults and children. The exercise program is uniquely adapted to each individual by the amount of resistance used.

Will my child's grades improve after we have done these exercises?

Writing, sitting still, and paying attention become easier for the child if the STNR exercises are done properly and sufficiently. Consequently, schoolwork generally improves.

My child never crawled, but is making straight A's. Are these exercises necessary?

Some children make good grades in spite of STNR interference, but always at the expense of extra effort and energy. Maturing the reflex through these exercises obviously cannot significantly raise grades that are already good. However, the same good grades will be achieved more quickly and easily after maturing the STNR. (Even good teachers and parents often forget that schoolwork should be relatively easy for children of average ability or better.)

Why can my child's writing be so good sometimes and just terrible at other times?

It's estimated that the immature STNR makes writing tasks at least ten times harder. Consequently, a two-page assignment becomes the equivalent of twenty pages in effort and energy for an STNR child. If a child "bites the bullet" and works *really* hard, s/he may occasionally produce a very good paper. However, it is nearly impossible for anyone to work ten times harder than everyone else for an extended period of time.

Your book says STNR children should have to do only 10 percent of writing assignments themselves. Isn't that unfair to other students?

Because an immature STNR makes writing at least ten times harder, 10 percent of an assignment for an STNR student would be the equivalent of 100 percent of the effort and energy required of other students.

Won't other students resent that STNR kids are doing less work?

Most children are very accepting of other children's doing work at their own ability level. Most children like for other children to be successful so long as it doesn't take away from their own success. It has been our experience that the only children who complain about accommodations being made for STNR children are the ones who need, but are not receiving, the same accommodations. Besides, we are recommending a reduction only in the amount of writing, not in the amount of learning. (See next question.)

Will the child learn the material if s/he is doing only 10 percent of the work?

We recommend that STNR children do only 10 percent of the *writing,* but 100 percent of the thinking. They can display their knowledge of the other 90 percent of their work by giving their answers orally into a tape recorder, to another student, to a teacher's aide, or to the teacher. A teacher has a much better chance of finding out what an STNR child actually knows by testing orally rather than through writing.

What can we do about our homework battles until we get the STNR matured through the exercises? The whole family ends up in tears every night.

We urge the parents to do 90 percent of the writing. The child is to do 100 percent of the thinking, but only 10 percent of the writing. Explain to the teacher that you will not do the thinking for the child. Homework wars will significantly decrease once you have removed the burden of writing for the child.

If I do 90 percent of his homework writing now, won't he expect me to do his writing forever?

No. When children can write more easily (after having done the STNR exercises), it will be quicker for them to think and write for themselves. Once the STNR is matured, children may need to be gradually eased into doing more of their own writing. They understandably may have developed an emotional mind-set against writing because of the extreme difficulty they have had with it.

In the early grades, how will an STNR child learn to write if he is doing only 10 percent of it?

We can assure you that most STNR children write very shabbily indeed, especially when required to practice extensively. They will be better able to maintain the energy and effort and control required for legible handwriting if presented with short writing assignments. It is better for the STNR child to write five acceptable R's than to poorly produce another fifteen. (Remember, the production of writing is ten times harder for the STNR child.) Allowing the STNR child to practice writing at the chalkboard, standing at a desk or countertop, or lying on the floor will also help circumvent the interfering effect of the immature STNR.

Since the "Back to Sleep" campaign started, many babies are spending most of their time on their backs. How will a baby ever learn to crawl if s/he is never on the stomach?

Babies need to spend a significant amount of time on their stomachs when they are awake and can be monitored. A new campaign, "Tummy to Play," has recently started to encourage parents to put babies on their stomachs. See our section on "Back to Sleep" in chapter 2.

Is there a video or DVD supplement to your book?

Yes. We have both VHS and DVD. The video is available in NTSC (USA) or PAL format. See page 186 for order information.

Can we do these exercises from just the video/DVD?

No, you cannot do the exercises from just the video/DVD. The video/DVD shows how the exercises should look, but does not explain the entire program. The book explains the rationale and describes the entire program, including directions on how to do the exercises and how to schedule them.

Can we do these exercises successfully from just the book?

Yes. Following the directions carefully in the book is a good way to successfully complete the exercise program. Using the video or DVD as a supplement to the book is an even better way of achieving success. You may also visit the Miriam Bender Achievement Center.

**If we come to the clinic, how long does the first session take
and are there follow-up sessions?**

The first session takes approximately half a day (three to four hours). We administer the STNR crawling test to confirm the presence of the immature reflex at the interfering level. We talk to the family extensively concerning the implications of the immature STNR and then train family members or friends to be crawling partners with the client. We train the client and the crawling partner(s) to do the beginning exercises, tailoring the exercises to each individual client. Ideally, the client and crawling partner(s) will return to the clinic approximately every six to eight weeks for reevaluations, enabling us to monitor the progress and modify the exercises. Reevaluations continue throughout the eight to ten months of the program and are extremely important in ensuring its success.

Where is the Miriam Bender Achievement Center?

The home office of the Miriam Bender Achievement Center is in Indianapolis, Indiana (USA). We are hoping to open clinics throughout the world.

**How can I become certified in the Miriam Bender Exercise
Program so that I can open a clinic in my city?**

Contact us at the clinic. See page 186 for contact information.

Results of a Study Putting the STNR Program in Action in an Elementary School

The goal of this project was to reduce ADHD behaviors in first through fifth grade students through maturation of the STNR. Ultimately, improvement is anticipated in academic areas. However, many of these research participants were *not* in academic distress to begin with. (The pre-testing in reading and math showed the average to be nearly at grade level or better for all grades, first through fifth.)

Teachers referred forty-eight students—first through fifth grade— who displayed the immature STNR (ADHD) characteristics. Twenty-four of these students were paired with sixth grade volunteers in a program designed to correct these problems by maturing the STNR using the crawling exercises outlined in this book. Multiple comparisons were made between the experimental group and a control group of twenty-four children.

This project was approved and supported by the school board of Mill Creek School Corporation; the superintendent, Don Stinson; the principal, Rob Neier; along with the school faculty of Mill Creek West Elementary School. The school counselor, Dee Kenworthy, organized the scheduling, with learning disabilities teacher Lynn

O'Connell and computer technology assistant Kathy Blake implementing the activities.

A list of ADHD and immature STNR characteristics was sent to first through fifth grade teachers at Mill Creek West Elementary School, in Amo, Indiana, a small community west of Indianapolis. Teachers were asked to refer for inclusion in the research project those students displaying the characteristics described on p. 7 in this book. The names of 85 children were submitted from a population of 245. It is noted, again, that many of these children were not in academic distress. Nevertheless, *all* of them demonstrated behavior characteristics of ADHD and immature STNR. Letters were then sent to parents of the 85 nominated students for permission to include their children in the research project. Fifty parents gave permission. Pre-testing was done with 50 students; post-testing was done with 48. Two children were unable to complete the program, leaving a total of 48 children to be divided into two groups, experimental and control, with 24 children in each group. All 48 students were administered the following tests at the beginning and the end of the study: The Bender Test for Symmetric Tonic Neck Reflex Maturity, achievement tests in reading and math, behavioral checklists (one completed by the classroom teacher, one by the parents, one by a disinterested observer), and the Test Of Variable Attention (TOVA). TOVA materials and analysis were donated by Dr. Lawrence Greenberg of the TOVA Foundation.

We tested all participants at the beginning of the study with the Bender Test for Symmetric Tonic Neck Reflex Maturity. The test results for the students were at varying levels, but all indicated significant interference from an immature STNR.

School personnel, under the direction of Dee Kenworthy, administered and scored the Iowa Test of Basic Skills for reading and math. The TOVA was administered by school personnel and analyzed by the TOVA Foundation. Separate Conners' Behavioral Checklists were completed by the participants' classroom teachers and by the parents. (The Conners' Behavioral Checklist is a standardized rating form of various behaviors.) A school-created behavioral checklist was completed by a disinterested observer. Sixth graders were asked to volunteer as helpers in the exercise program. Letters were sent to the parents of those sixth graders who volunteered, asking permission for these students to participate in the program. Thirty-two sixth-grade students volunteered to help in the study.

The forty-eight children—first through fifth grade—participating in the research program were matched as closely as possible according to grade level, gender, and test scores. As it was considered impossible to match children on all factors involved, we selected STNR, reading, and math scores for matching purposes. These students were then randomly assigned to the experimental and control groups.

Learning disabilities teacher Lynn O'Connell and computer technology assistant Kathy Blake had received three days' training toward certification in the Miriam Bender Exercise Program prior to implementing the program at their school. The program consists of five different exercises. We initially trained the sixth-grade volunteers to implement the Crawling I exercise with first- through fifth-grade participants in the experimental group, under the pleasant and adept supervision of O'Connell and Blake. We also trained O'Connell and Blake to do the rocking exercise with all participants. Participants and volunteers were excused from classes for fifteen minutes per day, five days a week, reporting to the gymnasium to do the exercises. We visited the school and evaluated the progress of the participants every six to eight weeks, modifying the exercises as necessary for each child and training the sixth-grade volunteers in Crawling Exercises II and III as appropriate. (Crawling Exercises II and III were added as the participants' improving coordination enabled them to perform the exercises effectively.)

All scheduling was masterfully arranged by Kenworthy, with very little disruption to regular activities. With the enthusiastic cooperation of all teachers, and Neier, Kenworthy, O'Connell, and Blake, the crawling exercises were acceptable to the participating students and to the general student body. All the students were excited when it was announced that we were presenting the design of the study at the eleventh European Conference of Neuro-developmental Delay in Children with Specific Learning Disabilities, held in March 1999, in Chester, England.

In a school setting, the exercise program is designed to be completed within a full school year, approximately nine months. Because this study did not commence until November 1998, ending in May 1999, the participants did not have time to advance to the final exercise by the end of the school year. Consequently, the last exercise, Crawling IV, was not assigned. Nor could the follow-up activities of gross motor and fine motor be implemented. Nevertheless, significant improvement was achieved in numerous areas, even though the program was not completed. (It is noted that we volunteered to train the parents of the twenty-four experimental participants in the final exercise [Crawling IV] so that they could complete the program over the summer at their homes. Parents of eighteen children received this training.)

Results

A variety of statistical tests were run on the data to determine if there was significant improvement from the pre-test to the post-test for either the experimental group or the control group on any of the tests. In addition, tests were run to determine if the experimental group scored significantly better than the control group on the posttests.

Dependent t-tests (statistical measurements) were run on all of the pre- and post-measures to determine significant differences. In the Conners' Behavioral Checklist, a lower score is better. The following were found to be significant improvements for the experimental group, but not for the control group.

EXPERIMENTAL GROUP	Pre Mean	Post Mean	t-value
Reading Raw Score	23.88	26.38	-2.576
Conners' Behavioral Checklist for Teachers Inattentive	14.21	11.29	2.568
Conners' Behavioral Checklist for Parents Conduct Problem	8.9565	7.5714	2.429

	Pre Mean	Post Mean	t-value
Conners' Behavioral Checklist for Parents Learning Problem	7.2174	5.9048	3.277
Conners' Behavioral Checklist for Parents Anxiety	4.2609	3.2644	3.376
Conners' Behavioral Checklist for Parents Anxiety Hyperactivity Index	16.3043	12.3333	4.121
Behavioral Checklist for Disinterested Observer #4	.6713	.6797	3.219
Behavioral Checklist for Disinterested Observer #8	.5316	0	2.304
RTQ1 (response time quarter 1)	566.78	492.30	2.299
RTQ2 (response time quarter 2)	614.17	529.04	2.610
RTH1 (response time first half)	589.22	510.13	2.488
TOVA-VART (total variability)	215.15	181.44	2.096

$p < .05$ (The probability of these scores being due to chance is significantly low.)

On the TOVA, the raw scores (RTQ1, RTQ2, RTH1, VART, CO%Q3, CO%Q4, CO%H2, Co%T, CO#TB, and CO%T) improve as the score decreases. The standard scores (CSSQ3, CSSQ4, CSSH2, CSST, and CSSTB) improve as the score increases. The TOVA-VART indicates that there was less variance in the response time for correct answers (or more consistency as a group in the time taken for correct responses) in the experimental group from pre-test to post-test. This indicates the probability that the experimental group's responses were less impetuous and that they could remain on task better, with more consistency.

The control group also had significant changes from the pre-test to the post-test commissions on the TOVA. (Commissions were pressings of the button when there was no stimulus.)

CONTROL GROUP	Pre Mean	Post Mean	t-value
CO%Q3 (percent of commissions Q3)	30.49	19.55	-2.43
CO%Q4 (percent of commissions Q4)	33.45	22.80	-2.31
CO%H2 (percent of commissions H2)	32.92	21.14	-2.34
CO%T (total percent of commissions)	10.78	5.49	-2.37
CSSQ3 (commission standard score Q3)	96	105.88	-2.58
CSSQ4 (commission standard score Q4)	97.79	109.21	-2.56
CSSH2 (commission standard score H2)	96.58	108.08	-2.63
CSST (total commission standard score)	98.04	108.04	-2.70

(The probability of these scores being due to chance is significantly low.)

We can logically theorize that, because the control group had not improved in attention, they were not effectively engaged in the task—thereby making fewer errors of commission (pressing the button when they should not).

A Wilcoxon Signed Rank Test, a non-parametric test for dependent means, was also used to test the Behavior Checklist for Disinterested Observer. This test was used because the Disinterested scores are at the interval level, which calls for a non-parametric test. The same significant differences were found using this test as the dependent t-test above.

EXPERIMENTAL GROUP	Pre Mean	Post Mean	Z-value
Behavioral Checklist for Disinterested Observer #4	.6713	.6797	-2.714
Behavioral Checklist for Disinterested Observer #8	.5316	0	-2.121

$p < .05$ (The probability of these scores being due to chance is significantly low.)

Item four indicates that children in the experimental group used their time more wisely. The results of item eight indicate that they (experimental group) blurt out answers less frequently.

The control group significantly improved on items six and thirteen. Item six referred to beginning a task before receiving directions; item thirteen referred to making unnecessary noises. Improvement would indicate that the children in this group, in later testing, did not start before instruction and made fewer noises. We can theorize, for six, that the control group improved in this area because they became more resistant to beginning assignments at all; while we cannot explain the artifact in thirteen (lessened noises), it is possible that the control group children were quieter in an effort to draw less attention to their being off task (while, at the same time, children in the experimental group might have been making more noise because of their efforts to remain on task). The Behavior Checklist for Disinterested Observer has twenty-five items; however, these four were the only ones to significantly change from the pre-test to the post-test.

The final test run was an independent t-test. It was conducted to determine significant differences between the post-test scores of the experimental group and the control group. Significant differences were found on the Bender Test for Symmetric Tonic Neck Reflex Maturity and the commissions part of the TOVA.

	Experimental	Control	t-value
Bender Test for Symmetric Tonic Neck Reflex Maturity	33.92	62.83	-10.778
CO#TB (total number of commissions)	31.1739	17.5417	2.466
CO%T (total % of commissions)	9.839	5.491	2.502
CSSTB (total commission standard score)	93.9565	108.0417	-2.755

$P < .05$ (The probability of these scores being due to chance is significantly low.)

No other significant differences were found. The sample size for this experiment was quite small; it is probable that a larger sample size would have resulted in more significant differences.

Data were analyzed by Courtney Brown, Ph.D., Purdue University.

Discussion

The results of these tests indicate that the experimental group (students who did the crawling exercises) improved significantly in eleven factors. The control group (no exercises) improved significantly in only three areas and even those are open to interpretation.

The significant improvement in eleven areas is of major importance to educators:

1. maturation of the Symmetric Tonic Neck Reflex
2. reading raw score
3. attention
4. conduct
5. learning
6. less anxiety
7. less hyperactivity
8. less impulsivity
9. less wasting of class time
10. less blurting out answers
11. more consistency in response time on TOVA

Of major importance is the statistically significant improvement of the experimental group as compared to the control group on the Bender Test for Symmetric Tonic Reflex Maturity. This significant improvement for the experimental group indicates a maturation of the Symmetric Tonic Neck Reflex as a direct result of the crawling exercises, effected within a school site.

Difficulties in the ten other areas that showed significant improvement are usually cited in the diagnosis of ADHD. These problems are also symptomatic of an immature STNR. Consequently, the results of this study support the hypothesis that the maturation of the STNR is directly responsible for the significant improvements in all eleven areas within the experimental group.

Conclusion

This research presents and statistically supports a significantly effective, drug-free remediation for the reduction of ADHD behaviors. It also holds great promise for improvement in academic areas: the reading raw score significantly improved despite the facts that 1) the crawling program was not completed due to time limitations; and 2) academic distress was not a necessary criterion for inclusion in the study (pre-testing showed the average to be nearly at grade level or better for all the grades). The study also presents a model program available to all schools for remediation of the immature STNR, thereby presenting a drug-free program for reducing ADHD behaviors and very likely improving academic achievement.

This research demonstrates that such a program can be effectively implemented within a school setting. Prior to receiving the results of this study, Mill Creek West Elementary School personnel were so pleased with the observable improvements in the behavior and attention of the students in the experimental group that they implemented the program for those students in the control group.

Here are just a few of the many positive comments from parents and teachers concerning this crawling program for the maturation of the STNR:

A parent wrote the following note to Mrs. Kenworthy regarding the participation of her son in the school STNR study:

"————is much better at being able to sit still now. Since he participated in the STNR group and completed his crawling exercises, he has definitely shown improvement in his schoolwork. It is amazing how much these exercises have increased his ability to concentrate.

He seems to be much better at finishing thoughts and following through with ideas. Before, he would often become 'sidetracked' and not finish what he had started. *Thank you* for letting him crawl."

Another parent wrote, "———— doesn't seem to be as fidgety while watching TV. I don't see her sitting upside down in the recliner."

One of the teachers wrote, "———— coordination has improved. This was verified by the OT. His organizational skills are excellent this year. His behavior is much improved over last year as well."

The authors thank the school board of Mill Creek School Corporation; the administration and staff and students of Mill Creek West Elementary School; Dr. Courtney Brown, our statistician; and Dr. Lawrence Greenberg, of the TOVA Foundation, for their invaluable contributions to this study. School administrators or teachers who would like information about establishing a program to mature the STNR in their schools should contact the authors.

Glossary

ADHD (attention-deficit/hyperactivity disorder—often still referred to by some professionals as ADD/ADHD). The current label for a child's difficulty with maintaining attention or focus with or without hyperactivity. Other terms that have been used are *brain damage, brain dysfunction, hyperactivity, hyperkinesis,* and *short attention span.*

Crawling. A term often used by child-development specialists to mean the locomotion done with the belly on the floor. The term *creeping* is usually used when the baby's belly is up off the floor and there is a "box" area of space. However, the general public uses the term *crawling* for the motion with the belly up off the floor, so we have used the term this way in our book.

Creeping. See Crawling.

Directionality. The external, or "out in space" awareness of "sided-ness." A good sense of directionality helps a child recognize quickly, without having to figure it out, the difference between *b* and *d* and *was* and *saw* and which is left and which is right.

Dysgraphia. Extreme difficulty with the physical aspect of writing. Our clinical experience has convinced us that this difficulty with writing is often due to the discomfort caused by an immature STNR rather than to a neurological inability to produce words.

Dyslexia. A term originally used to mean extreme difficulty with words or reading. Now it is used so indiscriminately that it is sometimes called a "garbage can" term (a term used for anything) and is used for everything from troubles with spelling to troubles with tying shoes.

Fine motor. The highest and last to develop of the motor skills, those that use the smaller muscles, e.g., writing, coloring.

Gross motor. The first to develop of the motor skills, those that use the larger muscles, e.g., running, throwing, kicking.

Hyperactivity. Purposeless overactivity.

Laterality. The internal awareness of "sidedness." A good sense of laterality leads to quick awareness of direction. A basic component of the development of laterality is proper, sufficient crawling.

Learning disability. A general or specific difficulty with a motor or academic task in a person of average or better-than-average intelligence. A significant discrepancy between a person's intellectual potential and that person's performance is usually caused by a learning disability.

Reversals. Writing or printing letters or numbers backward or upside down; writing or saying a number or word backward, e.g., *saw* for *was* or *51* for *15*.

STNR. Symmetric tonic neck reflex, an automatic movement (reflex) that develops when a child is between four and eight months of age. When this reflex is not integrated (matured) through proper and sufficient crawling, the immature reflex contributes to discomfort, poor attention, and poor coordination, especially in tasks such as writing.

References

ADHD.com. Medication used to treat ADHD and related disorders (2003). Retrieved October 29, 2003, from http://www.adhd.com/treat/med.html.

Anderson, R. *First Steps to a Physical Basis of Concentration*. Wales: Crown House Publishing, Ltd.; (1999).

Anselmo, S., and Franz, W. *Early childhood development: prenatal through age eight*. Englewood Cliffs, NJ: Prentice-Hall; (1995).

Audio-Digest family practice. ADHD 51(2003)(18).

Ayres, A. J. Improving academic scores through sensory integration. *Journal of Learning Disabilities* 5:342 (1972).

Balch, P. and J. Balch. *Prescription for Nutritional Healing*. New York: Avery; (2000).

Barsch, R. H. *Learning disabilities—a statement of position*. Washington, DC: Division for Children with Learning Disabilities (1967).

———. *Achieving perceptual motor efficiency*. Vol. 1. Seattle: Special Child Publications (1968).

Bender, M. L. A study of the relationships between persistent immaturity of the symmetric tonic neck reflex and learning disabilities in children. Ph.D. diss., Purdue University. (1971).

———. *The Bender-Purdue reflex test and training manual*. San Rafael, CA: Academic Therapy Publications (1976).

———. Interview with authors. (1997).

Bobath, K., and B. Bobath. Tonic reflexes and righting reflexes in the diagnosis and assessment of cerebral palsy. *Cerebral Palsy Review* 16 (1955): 4–10.

————. The neurodevelopmental treatment of cerebral palsy. *Journal of the American Physical Therapy Association* 47:(1967)11–14.

Center for the Advancement of Health. "Back to sleep" may slow development of head control (2001). Retrieved October 22, 2001, from http://www.cfah.org/hbns/newsrelease/back10-11-01.cfm.

Cook, P. The relationship of Bender facilitating exercises to ocular control and to achievement test scores. Ph.D. diss., Purdue University (1973).

Crook, W. *Help for the Hyperactive Child*. Jackson, TN: Professional Books; (1991).

Cruickshank, W. M. *Psychology of Exceptional Children*. Englewood Cliffs, NJ: Prentice-Hall; (1963).

————, and G. O. Johnson, eds. *Education of Exceptional Children and Youth*. 2d ed. Englewood Cliffs, NJ: Prentice-Hall; (1967).

Della Valle, J. An experimental investigation of the relationship(s) between preference for mobility and the word recognition scores of seventh-grade students to provide supervisory and administrative guidelines for the organization of effective instructional environments. Ph.D. diss., St. John's University; (1984).

Dennison, P. and G. Dennison. *Brain Gym*. Ventura, CA: Edu-Kinesthetics, Inc.; (1986).

Diagnostic and Statistical Manual of Mental Disorders: DSM-IV-TR. Washington, DC: American Psychiatric Association; C2000.

Dillon, E. J., E. J. Heath, and C. W. Biggs. *Comprehensive programming for success in learning*. Columbus, OH: Charles E. Merrill; (1970).

Dunn, K., and R. Dunn. Dispelling outmoded beliefs about student learning. *Educational Leadership* (March 1987):56–62.

Early, G. H. *Perceptual Training in the Curriculum*. Columbus, OH: Charles E. Merrill; (1969).

————, E. J. Heath, and M. L. Bender. Developing perceptual-motor skills—motor and reflex evaluations: Some new insights. *Academic Therapy* 6(1971):413–416.

Executive Parent.com. Your crawling 8-month-old (2003). Retrieved October 20, 2003, from http://executiveparent.com/cgi-bin/SoftCart.exe/ages 0-3yrs/article10.

Fiorentino, M. *Reflex Testing Methods for Evaluating C. N. S. Development*. Springfield, IL: Charles C. Thomas; (1963).

————. *Normal and abnormal development: The influence of primitive reflexes on motor development*. Springfield, IL: Charles C. Thomas; (1972).

Flax, N. Visual function in learning disabilities. *Journal of Learning Disabilities* 1:33–37; (1968).

Foundation for the study of infant deaths. Sleep on the back, play on the front, sit up and watch the world (2000). Retrieved January 13, 2003, from http://www.sids.org.uk/fsid/babiesruspr.htm.

Freides et al. Blind evaluation of body reflexes and motor skills in learning disability. *Journal of Autism and Developmental Disorders* 10 (1980).

Frostig, M. *Developmental test of visual perception: administration and scoring manual*. Palo Alto, CA: Psychologists Press; (1966).

Fysh, P. Late walkers are naturally smarter (2003). *ChiroWeb*. Retrieved October 20, 2003, from http://www.chiroweb.com/archives/13/12/20.html.

Gardner, A. "Back to sleep" campaign has curious side effect. *The Stress of Life* (2003). Retrieved October 20, 2003, from http://thestressoflife. com/back_to_sleep_campaign_has_curio.htm.

Gilbert, A. Brain dance for babies. *La Leche League International* (2001). Retrieved October 20, 2003, from http://www.llli.net/NB/NBMarApr01p44.html.

Gillette, H. *Systems of therapy in cerebral palsy*. Springfield, IL: Charles C. Thomas; (1969).

Goddard, Sally. *Reflexes, Learning and Behavior*. Eugene, OR: Fern Ridge Press; 2002.

Gold, Svea. *If Kids Just Came with Instruction Sheets*. Eugene, OR: Fern Ridge Press; 1997.

Gruber, J. J. Implications of physical education programs for children with learning disabilities. *Journal of Learning Disabilities* 2(1969): 593–599.

Hagan, N. Back to sleep—tummy to play: guidelines for infants. *Meriter Healthy Living*. Retrieved February 6, 2003, from http://www.meriter. com/living/Library/parent/backto.htm.

Halgren, M. R. Opus in see sharp. *Education* 81(1961):369–371.

Hannaford, Carla. *Smart Moves*. Arlington, VA: Great Ocean Publishers, Inc.; (1995).

Hebb, D. O. *The organization of behavior*. New York: John Wiley & Sons; (1949).

———. *A textbook of psychology*. 2d ed. Philadelphia: W. B. Saunders; (1966).

Hellebrandt, F. A., M. Schade, and M. L. Carns. Methods of evoking the tonic neck reflexes in normal human subjects. *American Journal of Physiological Medicine* 41(1962):90–139.

Hodges, H. An analysis of the relationships among preferences for a formal/informal design, one element of learning style, academic achievement, and attitudes of seventh and eighth grade students in remedial mathematics classes in a New York City alternative junior high school. Ph.D. diss., St. John's University; (1985).

Ismail, A. H., and J. J. Gruber. *Motor Aptitude and Intellectual Performance*. Columbus, OH: Charles E. Merrill; (1967).

Itard, J. [1894] *Rapports et memoires sur le sauvage de L'Aveyron* (Wild Boy of Aveyron). Translated by C. and M. Humphrey. New York: Meredith; 1962.

Kephart, N. C. *Learning Disability: An Educational Adventure*. West Lafayette, IN: Kappa Delta Pi Press; 1968.

———. *The Slow Learner in the Classroom*. 2d ed. Columbus, OH: Charles E. Merrill; 1971.

Kinderstart. Developmental milestones: crawling. *Child Development* (2000). Retrieved October 20, 2003, from http://www.kinderstart.com/childdevelopment/crawling.html.

Kolata, G., and H. Markel. (April 29, 2001, *New York Times*.) Infants who skip crawling still normal, research finds. *Indianapolis Star*, Sec. A, 1.

Konishi, Y., M. Kuriyama, H. Mikawa, J. Suzuki. Effect of body position on later postural and functional lateralities of pre-term infants. *Developmental Medicine and Child Neurology*, 29 (1987):751–57.

Kornblau, B. Once upon a time, babies crawled. Letters to the Editor. *New York Times* (May 2, 2001).

Krippner, S. Research in visual training and reading disability. *Journal of Learning Disabilities* 4(1971):65–76.

Laidlow, R.W., and M. S. Hamilton. A study of thresholds in apperception of passive movement among normal subjects. *Bulletin of the Neurological Institute of New York* 6(1937):268–73.

Lerner, J. W. *Learning Disabilities: Theories, Diagnosis, and Teaching Strategies*. 6th ed. Boston: Houghton Mifflin; 1993.

———. *Learning Disabilities: Theories, Diagnosis, and Teaching Strategies*. 7th ed. Boston: Houghton Mifflin; 1997.

Loikith, C. Once upon a time, babies crawled. Letters to the Editor. *New York Times*. (May 2, 2001).

Loyd, G. Developmental neurobics (2003). Retrieved October 20, 2003, from http://www.developmentalmovement.org/neurobics.htm.

McCormick, C. C., J. N. Schnobrich, S. W. Footlik, and B. Poetker. Improvement in reading achievement through perceptual-motor training. *Research Quarterly* 39(1968):627–33.

McGee, L. Back to sleep, prone to play. *e The Health Magazine for You*. (Fall 2001.) Retrieved January 13, 2003, from http://www.erlanger.org/e-magazine/Fall2001/sleep.htm.

McGraw, M. *The Neuromuscular Maturation of the Human Infant*. New York: Haefner; 1963.

Merton, P. A. How we control the contraction of our muscles. *Scientific American* 226 (no. 5)(1972):30–37.

Milani-Comparetti, A., and E. Gidoni. Pattern analysis in motor development and its disorders. *Developmental Medicine and Child Neurology* 9(1967a):625–30.

———. Routine developmental examination in normal and retarded children. *Developmental Medicine and Child Neurology* 9(1967b): 631–38.

Miller, J. *Your Child Needs a Champion*. Lebanon, PA: JMA Publications; 1997.

Milner, P. M. *Physiological Psychology*. New York: Holt, Rinehart & Winston; 1970.

O'Connor, C. Effects of selected physical activities upon motor performance, perceptual performance and academic achievement of first graders. *Perceptual and Motor Skills* 29(1969):703–09.

O'Dell, N. A study of the relationship of Bender resisted exercises to the symmetric tonic neck reflex and to achievement test scores. Ph.D. diss., Purdue University (1973).

Physicians' Desk Reference. 57th Edition. Montvale, NJ:Thomson PDR; 2003.

Piaget, J. *The Origins of Intelligence in Children*. New York: International Universities Press, Inc.; 1952.

———. *Science of Education and the Psychology of the Child*. New York: Orion Press; 1970.

Pontius, K., M. Aretz, C. Griebel, C. Jacobs, K. LaRock, & members of the OT-PT Baby Team. Back to sleep—tummy time to play. *The Newsletter of the Children's Hospital Physical Medicine and Rehabilitation, P M & R Update*, 4 (4)(2001), Denver, CO: Department of Rehabilitation at the Children's Hospital.

Porretto, D. Go, baby, go! *american baby*, LXV (1)(2003):47–50.

Professional's Guide to Patient Drug Facts. St. Louis: Facts and Comparisons—A Wolters Kluwer Co.; 1995.

Russell, D. H. *Children's Thinking*. Boston: Ginn; 1956.

Ryan, K., and J. Cooper. *Those Who Can, Teach*. Boston: Houghton Mifflin; 1995.

Sapir, S. *Learning Disability and Deficit Centered Classroom Training*. New York: Columbia University; 1969.

Seiderman, A. S. Motor planning and developmental apraxia. *Journal of the American Optometric Association* 41(1970):846–57.

Shea, T. C. An investigation of the relationship among preferences for the learning style element of design, selected instructional environments, and reading achievement of ninth grade students to improve administrative determinations concerning effective educational facilities. Ph.D. diss., St. John's University (1983).

Solan, H. A., and A. S. Seiderman. Case report on a grade one child before and after perceptual-motor training. *Journal of Learning Disabilities* 3(1970):635–39.

Steinhaus, A. The role of motor activity in mental and personality development. Report presented at symposium on integrated development, Purdue University (June 1964).

Stevens, L. J. *12 Effective Ways to Help Your ADD/ADHD Child.* New York: Avery; 2000.

Strauss, A. A., and L. E. Lehtinen. *Psychopathology and Education of the Brain-Injured Child.* New York: Grune & Stratton; 1947.

Swiatek, J. (2004, March 23.) FDA urges warning on antidepressants. *Indianapolis Star,* Sec. A, 1.

U.S. Department of Health, Education, and Welfare, National Project on Learning Disabilities in Children. *Minimal brain dysfunction in children.* Public Health Service Publication No. 2015. Washington, DC: U.S. Government Printing Office (1969).

Watson, L. The other side of "Back to Sleep." *Epinions* (2002). Retrieved January 13, 2003, from http://www.epinions.com/kifm-review-47E-460BD462-3A4D5FOB-prod3.

White, B. L. *The First Three Years of Life.* New York: Prentice-Hall; 1990.

Whitehead, A. N. *The Aims of Education.* New York: The New American Library; 1957.

Young, F. A., and D. B. Lindsley, eds. *Early Experience and Visual Information Processing in Perceptual and Reading Disorders.* Washington, DC: National Academy of Sciences (1970).

Index

Note: *Italic* numbers indicate illustrations.

Academic achievement, xv
    immature STNR and, 54, 94, 98
    STNR exercises and, 216–19
Academic problems, 37
    misdiagnosis, 72–73
    physicians and, 34
    STNR and, 33, 69, 71–72, 125
Accelerated classes, 94–96
ADD (Attention Deficit Disorder). *See*
    ADHD
Adderall, Adderall XR (amphetamine),
    189–90
ADHD (Attention-Deficit Hyperactivity
    Disorder), xvii, 1, 36, 205, 231
    in adults, 4, 10
    immature STNR and, 3–5, 70
    medication for, 35, 187–89
        STNR exercises and, 216
    typical behaviors, 7–8, 9–11
        STNR exercises and, 229
    See also STNR (Symmetric Tonic Neck
    Reflex)
ADHD students, study of, 222–30
Adults
    ADHD diagnosis, 4, 10
    STNR exercises for, 216
After-school behavior, 114
Age for STNR exercises, 136, 206–7, 208
Aggression, immature STNR and, 62, 210
Agitation, 203
Alopecia (hair thinning), 203
    drug side effect, 199

Amphetamine (Adderall, Adderall XR),
    189–90
Anderson, R., 69
Anorexia, 203
Anselmo, S., 16
Antianxiety medications, side effects,
    200–201
Anticonvulsants, side effects, 198–99
Antidepressants, side effects, 193–98
Antihypertensive medications, side effects,
    192–93
Anti-mania medications, side effects, 202
Antipsychotics, side effects, 201–2
Appetite loss, drug side effect, 189, 192, 199
Arithmetic, problems of, 71
Arms, reaching positions, 40–41, *41*
Arm Twirls exercise, 178
"Army crawl," 31
Arrhythmia, 203
Art classes, 90–91
Arthralgia (joint pain), 203
Asthenia (weakness), 203
Asymmetric Tonic Neck Reflex (ATNR),
    211
Ataxia, 203
Athletic activities, avoidance of, 7
Athletic skills, poor, 9, 130
Ativan (lorazepam), 200–201
ATNR (asymmetric tonic neck reflex), 211
Atomoxetine HCL (Strattera), 192
Attention-deficit/hyperactivity disorder. *See*
    ADHD

Attention problems, 7–8, 9, 52, 69, 130
  circumventions, 67
  sitting comfort and, 73–74
  STNR and, 70, 71
Autistic children, 210
Automatic movement, infant reflex, 16
  STNR, 18–32
Automatic reaction, reflex as, 17
Automobiles, discomfort in, 119–20
Avoidance, 61–62, 66, 125
Awkward movements, 7, 9, 130
Ayers, Jean, 72

Babinski reflex, 16
"Back to Sleep" movement, 26–29, 219
Balance
  poor, drug side effect, 200
  STNR and, 85, 103
Balancing exercise, 179
Barbershops, problems in, 123
Baseball, 100–102
Basketball, 102
Beauty salons, problems in, 123
Behavioral checklists, ADHD research
        program, 222, 224–27
Behavioral problems, 7–8, 9–11
  drug therapy, 35
  educators and, 35–37
  at home, 110–18
  misdiagnosis, 72–73
  in public settings, 119–27
  at school, 69–98
  STNR and, 33, 50–53, 94, 125, 130
Behavior modification, 38
Bender, Miriam L., vii, xvii-xviii, 18, 23, 58,
        65, 71, 78, 129, 143, 185
  and crawling, 22
  foreword, xv-xvi
  and learning disabilities, 3–5, 31
  STNR test, 134
Bender Test for STNR Maturity, 222, 227
  experimental group improvement, 228
Bicycle riding, difficulty of, 60–61
Biggs, C. W., 22
Blake, Kathy, 222, 223
Blame, for children's problems, 37
Blinking reflex in infants, 17
Blythe, 85
Body, control of, STNR and, 69
Body language, STNR and, 50–53
Body position, for writing, 181–83, 182,
        183
"Boredom," of gifted students, 95

Box position, 141–42, 142, 145, 147, 150,
        154, 157, 164–65, 171
Brain Gym, Dennison and Dennison, 177
Brown, Courtney, 228, 230
Bupropion (Wellbutrin), 198
BuSpar (buspirone), 201

"Camel walk," 31
Carbamazepine (Tegretol), 199
Cars, discomfort in, 119–20
Casts on legs, in infancy, 26, 130
Catapres (clonidine), 193
Catching a ball, 100–101
Cat sit position, 20, 20, 22, 105
Celexa (citalopram hydrobromide), 193,
        194
Center for the Advancement of Health, 26
Chair tipping, 42–43
Chalkboard, for writing exercises, 180
Chalkboard work, as circumvention, 97
Childhood development, early, 15–18
Children
  with ADHD, medication of, 187–89
  with immature STNR, 66, 73, 209–19
    academic problems, 3–5
    home problems, 110–18
    in public settings, 119–27
    school problems, 69–98
    and sports, 99–109
Circumventions, 65–67, 125
  attention-span improvement, 74–75
  at home, 111–17
  in public settings, 120–24, 126–27
  at school, 83–84, 88, 89–90, 91, 93–97
Citalopram hydrobromide (Celexa), 193,
        194
Clonidine (Catapres), 193
Clothing, for crawling exercises, 135
Clumsiness, 7, 9, 52, 57, 130
  drug side effect, 200
Cognitive function, crawling and, 23
Coloring, in art class, 90
Computer, for writing problem, 84, 97
Concerta (methylphenidate), 190
Constipation, drug side effect, 192, 193, 200
Cook, Patricia A., xv-xvi, xx
Cooper, J., 95
Cooperative games, 116
Coordination, 15–18, 108–9
  exercises to improve, 177–84
  poor, 52
    and athletic performance, 99
    immature STNR and, 92–94, 103–5

Coping mechanisms, circumventions, 66
Correct sitting position, 70
Coughing reflex, in infants, 17
Crawling, xvii, 2, 85, 206, 231
  and directionality, 86–87
  inadequate, 29–32, 130, 207, 209–10
    and math problems, 89
    reasons for, 25–29
  and motor development, 27–29
  position for, 21, 21, 22
  and sequencing, 88
  and STNR, 21–24
  See also STNR exercises
Crawling exercises, school research pro-
    gram, 221–30
  See also STNR exercises
Creeping, 21n. See also Crawling
Cross-lateral movements, 23
Cursive writing, exercises, 180–84
Cylert (pemoline), 190

Daydreaming, 7, 9, 52, 79, 130
Defense mechanisms, 125
Della Valle, J., 51
Dennison, G., 177
Dennison, P., 177
Dentists, visits to, 122
Depakote (divalproex sodium), 199
Depth perception, STNR and, 85
Desipramine (Norpramin), 195
Developmental milestone, crawling as,
    27–28
Dexedrine (dextroamphetamine), 190
Dexmethylphenidate hydrochloride (Fo-
    calin), 191
Dextrostat (dextroamphetamine sulfate),
    190
Diarrhea, drug side effect, 193
Dietary changes, 207
Dillon, E. J., 22
Directionality, 29–30, 52, 86–87, 231
  poor, and dyslexia, 86
Discipline, 37–38
  poor, immature STNR and, 119
Discomfort, physical
  of ADHD children, 11–14
  immature STNR and, 8, 9
  from STNR exercises, 137
Disruptive behaviors, 7–8, 9–11
Divalproex sodium (Depakote), 199
Dizziness, drug side effect, 192, 200
Doctor's office, problems in, 122–23
Drawing, 90

Drowsiness, drug side effect, 192, 200, 201
Drug therapy, for ADHD children, 35,
    187–89
  potential side effects, 189–202
Dunn, Kenneth, 51
Dunn, Rita, 51
Duration of exercises
  gross motor exercises, 177
  STNR exercises, 129, 136
    Crawling I, 152, 156
    Crawling II, 161–62
    Crawling III, 168–69
    Crawling IV, 174
    Resisted Rocking, 148
  writing exercises, 183, 184
Dyscalculia (math difficulty), 88–90
Dysgraphia, 231
  See also Writing, problems of
Dyslexia, 84–88, 232
Dyspepsia, 203
Dysphoria, 203
Dyspnea, 203

Early, G. H., 22
Educators, and behavior problems, 35–37
Effexor (venlafaxine), 193, 194
Efficiency, directionality and, 86
Effort requirements, STNR and, 58, 60, 66,
    71, 73, 77, 78–80, 217–19
  for motor skill development, 108–9
  at school, 114
  for writing, 4
Elavil (amitriptyline), 194
Elbows, in exercise modifications, 163, 164,
    169–70, 170
Elementary school, STNR program,
    221–30
Emory University, STNR study, 51, 72
Emotional problems, immature STNR and,
    33, 47, 54
Energy expenditure, STNR and, 71
Enrichment classes, 94–96
Environmental factors
  in immature STNR, 208
  in inadequate crawling, 25–26
Epistaxis, 203
Escitalopram oxalate (Lexapro), 195
Eskalith (lithium carbonate), 202
Euphoria, 203
European Conference of Neuro-develop-
    mental Delay in Children with
    Specific Learning Disabilities, 223
Executive Parent, 28

Exercises to improve coordination, 177–84
  See also STNR exercises
Exfoliative dermatitis, 203
Eye control, STNR exercises and, 213
Eye examinations, problems with, 122
Eyes, training of, STNR and, 85

Family activities, problems with, 115–16, 124
Fatigue
  drug side effect, 192
  of STNR children, after-school, 114
Field, Jane, 69
Fine-motor coordination, 16, 232
  in drawing, 90–91
  exercises to improve, 179–84
Flax, N., 22
Fluoxetine (Prozac), 196–96
Fluvoxamine (Luvox), 195
Focalin (dexmethylphenidate hydrochloride), 191
Focusing of eyes, STNR and, 85
Football, 103–4
Foot positions, in STNR children, 2–3, 43–44, 44, 70
Foot Touch exercise, 178
Foundation for the Study of Infant Deaths, 27
Franz, W., 16
Freides et al., 51, 72
Frequency of exercises
  gross motor exercises, 177
  STNR exercises, 136, 215
    Crawling I, 152, 156
    Crawling II, 161
    Crawling III, 168
    Crawling IV, 174
    Resisted Rocking, 148
  writing exercises, 183, 184
Frostig, M., 22
Frustration, immature STNR and, 60–64
Fysh, P., 28

Gag reflex, 17
Games, family recreation, 115–16
Gardner, A., 27
Genetic factors in STNR problems, 25, 208
Gidoni, E., 21
Gifted children, STNR and, 94–95
Gilbert, A., 28, 129
Glycosuria, 203
Goalie, in hockey, 106–7

Goddard, Sally, 85, 133
Gold, S., 37
Golf, 108
Grasping reflex, 16
Greenberg, Lawrence, 222, 230
Gross-motor coordination, 16, 232
  exercises to improve, 177–79
  STNR and, 208–9
Group activities, 62
Growth, lack of, drug side effect, 189
Guanfacine (Tenex), 193

Hagan, N., 27
Hair loss, drug side effect, 199
Hand-eye coordination, STNR and, 85
Hand position, in STNR exercises, 213
  in exercise modifications, 163, 164, 169–70, 170
"Hangover effect," drug side effect, 200
Hannaford, Carla, 23, 24
Head
  control of, by infants, 19, 26
  flattened (plagiocephaly), 27
  position in STNR exercises, 212, 213
    Crawling I exercise, 150, 151, 152, 154, 155, 155
    Crawling II exercise, 157, 157, 160–61, 169–70
    Crawling III exercise, 165, 167
    Crawling IV exercise, 171, 173
    Resisted Rocking exercise, 144, 145, 146, 148
  resting position, 45, 45
Headache
  drug side effect, 189, 193, 198, 200
  immature STNR and, 41–42
Heath, E. J., 22
Hockey, 106–7
Hodges, H., 51
Home behaviors, 11, 110–18
Homework, 52, 112–14, 218
  time spent on, 75–77
Hyperactivity, 232
Hypertension, 203
Hyperthermia, 203
Hypertonia, 203
Hyperventilation, 203
Hypesthesia, 203

Imipramine (Tofranil), 197
Inattentiveness, 79
Indianapolis Star, 27
Individual activities, 62

Infants
  encouragement to crawl, 206, 207
  newborn, reflexes, 16–18
Inflexibility, 62–64
Info for Living (TV program), xviii
Insomnia, 203
  drug side effect, 189, 193, 198
Intelligence
  crawling and, 30
  and directionality, 86
  immature STNR and, 54, 94
Interactions between medications, 189
Interfering effects of immature STNR,
      69–70, 72–74, 108–9
  writing problems, 75–83, *81, 82*
Interventions, 65
  See also STNR exercises
Involuntary action, reflex as, 17
  STNR, 2
Iowa Test of Basic Skills, 222
Ipsilateral crawling pattern, 171, 215
Irritability, drug side effect, 189
Irritating behavior, 111

Keller, Helen, xx
Kenworthy, Dee, 221, 222, 223
Kephart, Newell C., xviii, 22
Kicking exercise, 179
Kinderstart, 28
Knees, protection for, 135, 216
Konishi, Y., 26

Large muscle movement, 16
Laterality, 29–30, 232
Laziness, appearance of, 34, 55, 57, 71–72,
      78, 95
Learning, 18
  enhancement of, 129
Learning disability, 232
  immature STNR and, 3–5, 51
  inadequate crawling and, 24, 31
Learning disabled children, work with,
      xviii
Leg braces, in infancy, 26, 130
Lerner, J. W., 31
Letters, reversal of, 7, 9, 30, 84–86, 130
Lexapro (escitalopram oxalate), 194, 195
Lithium carbonate (Eskalith), 202
Locomotion, alternative forms, 31
Loikith, C., 28
Lorazepam (Ativan), 200–201
Loyd, G., 27, 28
Luvox (fluvoxamine), 194, 195

McGee, L., 27
Mania, 203
Math, difficulty with, 88–90
Maturity of STNR, 21–24, 125, 187, 209
  test for, 174–76
  See also STNR; STNR exercises
Mealtimes, STNR and, 110–12
Medical profession, and STNR, 205–6
Medication of ADHD children, 187–89
Memory loss, drug side effect, 200
Merton, P. A., 143
Metadate ER (methylphenidate), 191
Methylphenidate:
  Concerta, 190
  Metadate ER, 191
  Ritalin, Ritalin SR, 191–92
  Ritalin LA, 192
Milani-Comparetti, A., 21
Mill Creek School Corporation, 221–30
Miller, J., 35
Milner, P. M., 143
Miriam Bender Achievement Center, 125,
      129, 130–31, 134, 220
Miriam Bender Exercise Program, 223
Mirtazapine (Remeron), 197
Misdiagnosis of STNR children, 33–34
Moodiness, drug side effect, 189
Mood swings, drug side effect, 192
Moro (startle) reflex in infants, 17
Motivation, lack of, 55, 57, 78, 108
Motor coordination, 15–18
  poor, and writing, 14
Motor development, early, xv, 72, 143
  crawling and, 27–29
Motor skills, inadequate, 55–57
  immature STNR and, 92–94, 108
Mouth, dry, drug side effect, 192
Movement
  frequent, 7, 9
  involuntary, 69
  space for, 126
Muscle stiffness, drug side effect, 201
Muscular spasms (tics), drug side effect,
      189
Muscular tension, immature STNR and,
      2–3, 69–70, 78
Music lessons, 91, 115
Myasthesia, 203
Myclonus, 203

Nausea, drug side effect, 189, 192, 200, 201
Neck muscles, back sleeping and, 26–27
Neck pain, in STNR exercises, 137, 212–13

Nefazodone hydrochloride (Serzone), 197
Neier, Rob, 221, 223
Nervousness, drug side effect, 193
Neural efficiency, resistance and, 143
New York Times, 27
Niebuhr, Reinhold, xx
Nightmares, drug side effect, 200
Nonphysical activities, 62
Non-stimulant drugs, side effects, 192
Norpramin (desipramine), 195
Nortriptyline (Pamelor), 195–96
Number reversals, 7, 9, 30, 84–86, 89, 130
Nystagmus, 204

O'Connell, Lynn, 221–22, 223
O'Dell, Nancy E., xv-xvi, xx, 22
Olanzapine (Zyprexa), 202
Orthostatic hypotension, 204
Overactivity, 34–35, 114
Overriding of reflexes, 18

Palpitations, 204
Pamelor (nortriptyline), 195–96
Parents, 37–38, 76–77, 98
    demands by, immature STNR and,
        60–61
    and STNR exercises, 135–37, 211
Paresthesia, 204
Paroxetine (Paxil), 196
Partners for exercises, 135–37
Patience needed, 97–98, 117
Pavlides, 85
Paxil (paroxetine), 194, 196
Peer relationships, poor, 54–57
Pemoline (Cylert), 190
Pencils, grip of, 79–80, 113
Photosensitivity, 204
Physical activities, 62
Physical education, STNR and, 92–94
Physical stress, STNR and, 78
Physicians
    and drug therapy, 187
    and STNR, 34–35, 205–6
Physicians' Desk Reference, 188
Piaget, J., 22
Plagiocephaly (flattened head), 27
Play, avoidance of, STNR and, 55–57
Playpens, 24, 25, 130, 207, 208
Pleasantness, of teachers, 97–98
Polyuria, 204
Pontius, K., 27
Porretto, D., 27
Positions, comfortable, circumventions, 66

Postural clues to immature STNR, 39–50
    body language, 50–53
Postural freedom, as circumvention, 74–75,
        96, 117
    at home, 111, 113, 115, 116, 117
    in public settings, 120, 122–26
    in school, 83, 88, 90, 91
Postures, inappropriate, 2–3, 9, 10–11
Prescription drugs, negative side effects,
        188–202
Professional's Guide to Patient Drug Facts,
        188
Proprioceptive feedback, 18, 30n, 143
Protective reactions in infants, 17
Prozac (fluoxetine), 194, 196–97
Pruritus, 204
Psychological interpretations of homework
        problems, 112–13
Psychological problems, immature STNR
        and, 54–64
Psychosis, 204
Public settings, problems in, 119–27
Purpura, 204

Reaching positions, 40–41, *41*
Reading, 84–88
    directionality and, 86
    posture and, 72
Reciprocal crawling pattern, 170–71, 215
Reclining position, 47–49, *48*
Recording of difficulties, 135
Reflexes, early, 15–18
Reflex stimulation/inhibition program,
        133
Religious services, problems, 121–22
Remeron (mirtazapine), 194, 197
Resistance, during exercises, 135
    maturity test, 175
    STNR exercises, 143, 214
        Crawling I, 151–52, 154, 155, 156
        Crawling II, 160
        Crawling III, 166
        Crawling IV, 172–73
Resisted Rocking exercise, 144–49, *144*,
        145, 146, 147, 154, 156, 161–62, *164,*
        168–69, 174
    32–week program, 138–40
Restaurants, problems in, 120–21
Reversals, 7, 9, 30, 84–86, 130, 232
    and math problems, 89
Reward for STNR exercises, 136
Rhythm of music, STNR and, 91
Risperidal (risperidone), 201–2

Ritalin, Ritalin LA, Ritalin SR
(methylphenidate), 191–92
Rocking exercise. *See* Resisted Rocking
exercise
Rooting reflex, 16
Running, 108
and catching, 93, 100–101
Ryan, K., 95

School, STNR program in, 221–30
School problems, 10–11, 69–96
general circumventions, 96–97
Seating arrangements, helpful, 111–12, 117,
120–21, 124, 126
Self-esteem, 67, 79, 111, 113, 118
STNR and, 58–60, 77
Sequencing, 87–88, 89
Sertraline (Zoloft), 198
Serzone (nefazodone hydrochloride), 194,
197
Shea, T. C., 51
Siblings, 210
and STNR exercises, 136–37
Side Bends exercise, 178
"Sidedness," 29–30, 86–87
Side effects of medications, 188–202
antianxiety, 200–201
anticonvulsant, 198–99
antidepressant, 193–98
antihypertensive, 192–93
anti-mania, 202
antipsychotic, 201–2
non-stimulant, 192
stimulant, 189–92
Side Twist exercise, 179
SIDS (sudden infant death syndrome), 26
Sitting, STNR and, 2–3, 7, 9–11, 69, 70
comfortable, circumventions for, 66
discomfort of, 38, 11–14, 39–50, 126
in art class, 90
and attention problems, 73–74
for homework, 112
at mealtimes, 111–12
in music class, 91
in travel, 119–20
inappropriate positions, 7–8, 52–53, 130
Skiing, 107
Sleep problems, drug side effects, 189, 193,
198, 200
Slouching posture, 2–3, 42, 43, 70
Small muscle movement, 16
Sneezing reflex, in infants, 17
Soccer, 108

Social demands, STNR and, 60–61
sports participation, 99
Social interactions, STNR and, 54–57
Somnolence, 204
Space perception, STNR and, 85
Space requirement for STNR exercises,
134–35, 216
Spectator events, problems at, 124
"Spelling Bee" exercise, 12, 13
Spelling problems, 71, 84–88
Sports, STNR and, 92–94, 99–109
avoidance of, 7, 9, 130
Squirming, 7, 9, 49–50, 130
Standing position, 46–47, 46
Startle reflex, in infants, 17
Step length, crawling exercises, 161, 162,
167, 167, 168
Stevens, L. J., 4
Stimulant medications, side effects, 189–92
Stinson, Don, 221
STNR (Symmetric Tonic Neck Reflex),
xvii, 15–32
immature, 1–3, 208–10, 232
circumventions, 65–67
and intelligence, 30, 94
interfering effects, 93, 98–109
interventions, 65
and learning disability, 31–32
postural clues, 39–50
public setting problems, 119–27
psychological consequences, 54–64
research project, 222
and school problems, 69–98
treatment approaches, 33–38
maturation of, 21–24, 125, 174–76, 187,
209, 211, 228–29
exercises for, 129, 133–34
See also STNR exercises
normal development, 24
test for, 134
relationship to reading, 85
STNR exercises, 129, 133–76, 212–16
age to begin, 206–7, 208
elementary school program, 221–30
Stomach, infant time on, 28–29
Stomach problems, drug side effects, 189,
192
Stopping Hyperactivity: A New Solution,
O'Dell and Cook, xviii-xix
Strattera (atomoxetine HCL), 192
Success, 58, 125
Sucking reflex, 16
Sudden infant death syndrome (SIDS), 26

Swallowing difficulty, drug side effect, 201
Swimming, 104–5
Symmetric Tonic Neck Reflex. *See* STNR

Tachycardia, 204
Targets, for crawling exercises, 135
 watching of, 213
Teachers, 40–42, 60–61, 97–98
 blaming of, 37
 and sitting positions, 2–3, 10, 52–53, 70
 and STNR children, 74–77, 80–82
 See also Circumventions
Teams, gym class, assignment to, 93
Teenagers, and STNR exercises, 210
Tegretol (carbamazepine), 199
Television, 116
Tenex (guanfacine), 193
Tennis, 108
Testing of students, research project, 222
Test of Variable Attention (TOVA), 222, 225, 227
Throwing a ball, 100–101
Tics, 204
 drug side effect, 189
Time requirements, STNR and
 for homework, 75–77
 for schoolwork, 55
 for writing, 4, 14, 71
Tinnitus, 204
Toe Touch exercise, 178
Tofranil (imipramine), 197
Torticollis (twisted neck), 27
TOVA. *See* Test of Variable Attention
Training for exercise programs, 186
Travel, problems with, 119–20

Tremor, 204
 drug side effect, 199
"Tummy to Play," campaign, 28–29, 219

Underachievement, STNR and, 94
Unsteadiness, drug side effect, 200
Urticaria, 204

Venlafaxine (Effexor), 194
Vertigo, 204
 drug side effect, 199
Visual skills, STNR and, 85
Volleyball, 103
Voluntary movements, 18
Vomiting, drug side effect, 192, 200

Walkers, 207–8
 and STNR, 24, 25
Walking, early, 24, 30, 94, 130
Wasting of time, 79
Watson, L., 27
Weight changes, drug side effect, 189, 193, 199
Wellbutrin (bupropion), 194, 198
White, B. L., 22–23
Wilcoxon Signed Rank Test, 226
Wrestling, 105–6, *105*
Writing problems, 3–4, 7, 9, 12–14, 38, 41, 52, 69, 70–71, 75–83, 81, 82, 95–96, 125, 130, 217–19
 circumventions, 67, 83–84, 96–97, 113
 directionality and, 86
 exercises to improve, 179–84, *180, 181, 182, 183*
 and math problems, 89

Zoloft (sertraline), 194, 198

About the Authors

Nancy E. Woodworth O'Dell received her bachelor of arts degree in English and her master's degree in education from Indiana University. She taught high school for two years and junior high school for two years before earning her Ph.D. from Purdue University, specializing in learning disabilities and child development, and working under the direction of Dr. Miriam Bender. She did school psychological evaluations and then went into private practice before becoming a professor at the University of Indianapolis. There, she taught classes in learning disabilities and child development. She also founded and codirected, with Dr. Patricia Cook, both the Miriam Bender Achievement Center and the Baccalaureate for University of Indianapolis Learning Disabled (B.U.I.L.D.), a support system for learning-disabled college students. She was named to the Warren Central High School Alumni Hall of Fame in 2002. She has given innumerable presentations about learning disabilities, especially about the symmetric tonic neck reflex and its implications for learning and behavior.

Patricia A. Cook received her bachelor of arts degree from Marian College in Indianapolis, majoring in English and biology. She earned her master's degree in educational psychology from Butler University while teaching high school English. She earned her Ph.D. from Purdue University, specializing in learning disabilities and educational psychology, and working under the guidance of Dr. Bender. She did school psychological testing, and then went into private practice with Dr. O'Dell before becoming a professor at the University of Indianapolis. With Dr. O'Dell, she founded and codirected the B.U.I.L.D. program and the Miriam Bender

Achievement Center. She was named Distinguished Alumnus of Marian College in 1986 and the *Indianapolis Star*'s Woman of the Year in 1988.

Now retired from the University of Indianapolis, both Drs. Cook and O'Dell are Professors Emeriti in the School of Education. They continue to promote and implement Dr. Bender's work at their Miriam Bender Achievement Center in Indianapolis, Indiana.

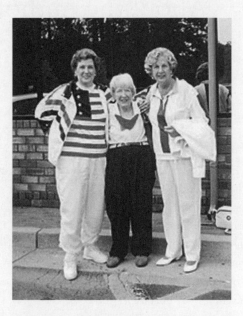

The authors with Miriam Bender (center)